£2.00

Bertie and Margaret

— every good wish
and love

5th August 1986

— the day of the
great reunion

Michael Howell
and Peter Ford

[signature]

Medical Mysteries

VIKING

VIKING
Penguin Books Ltd, Harmondsworth, Middlesex, England
Viking Penguin Inc., 40 West 23rd Street, New York, New York 10010, U.S.A.
Penguin Books Australia Ltd, Ringwood, Victoria, Australia
Penguin Books Canada Ltd, 2801 John Street, Markham, Ontario, Canada L3R 1B4
Penguin Books (N.Z.) Ltd, 182–190 Wairau Road, Auckland 10, New Zealand

First published 1985

Filmset in VIP Palatino
Typeset, printed and bound in Great Britain by
Hazell Watson & Viney Limited,
Member of the BPCC Group,
Aylesbury, Bucks

British Library Cataloguing in Publication Data

Howell, Michael
  Medical mysteries.
  1. Pathology—Case studies
  2. Wounds and injuries—Case studies
  I. Title   II. Ford, Peter, *1936*–
  616'.09   RB112

ISBN 0-670-80220-4

To our children

Simon, Mark, Matthew and Joanna
Piers, Julian and Isabel

and for the Matthew and Joanna
who are our friends

Contents

List of Plates

(Between pages 194 and 195)

(eds.), *Kuru: Early Letters and Field Notes from the Collection of D. Carleton Gajdusek*, Raven Press, New York, 1981)

13. A kuru patient in the disease's terminal stage (from Judith Farquhar and D. Carleton Gajdusek (eds.), *Kuru: Early Letters and Field Notes from the Collection of D. Carleton Gajdusek*, Raven Press, New York, 1981)

14. Scoular's cast of the skull of Robert the Bruce (Department of Anatomy, University Medical School, Edinburgh)

15. A reconstruction of King Robert's features, based on the cast of the skull (Department of Anatomy, University Medical School, Edinburgh)

16. Dr Møller-Christensen excavates a leper graveyard (courtesy of Dr Vilhelm Møller-Christensen)

17. A sequence of skulls showing progressive changes which leprosy may cause (prepared by Dr Ron Finch; courtesy of Dr Vilhelm Møller-Christensen)

18. Dr John Snow (Wellcome Institute for the History of Medicine)

19. Cartoon by John Leach: *A Court for King Cholera* (Wellcome Institute for the History of Medicine)

20. Sir Douglas Mawson (Mawson Institute for Antarctic Research, University of Adelaide)

21. The improvised tent used by Mawson (Mawson Institute for Antarctic Research, University of Adelaide)

22. Terrain of the kind faced by the Australian Antarctic Expedition of 1911–14 (Mawson Institute for Antarctic Research, University of Adelaide)

Introduction

The episodes selected for inclusion in this book may, on the whole, be better known to those who live within the world of medicine than to those who stand outside. We have therefore chosen stories which seem to justify retelling to a wider audience. These accounts contain their disasters and triumphs, their heroes and villains, both human and molecular. But the main purpose in telling a story should never be less than to engage and entertain, and any success which we may achieve in doing so needs to acknowledge the generous responses of others to appeals for information and the confirmation of facts. We are much in the debt of those who have given assistance with the episodes indicated.

'The Beetle of Aphrodite': Professor A. Polak of Portsmouth responded to a request for information; Dixon Scott searched out various press cuttings; John Wardman kindly commented on the pharmaceutical details; and Shelley Oakley provided a working translation from the French for the Heine article (cited in our sources).

'The Case of the Epping Jaundice': Dr Harry Kopelman, Dr Isidore Ash, Dr M. H. Robertson and Mr P. G. Sanders gave us an afternoon and their personal guidance through the intricacies of this fascinating incident.

'A Fallen Splendour': Dixon Scott again delved for relevant

press cuttings; and John Wardman again checked on our pharmaceutical assumptions.

'The Head that Wore a Crown': Professor G. J. Romanes of the Department of Anatomy, University of Edinburgh, granted us access to the cast of the skull alleged to be that of Robert the Bruce, provided photographs and allowed us to reproduce them; Professor Vilhelm Møller-Christensen was generous with his advice and also gave us permission to reproduce photographs; Dr Babette Evans of the Department of History, University of Leicester, read the final text and proffered valued advice on several historical details.

'The Stranded Eagle': Dr Holger Madser of Copenhagen was consistent in his interest and made many helpful suggestions as well as providing much information; the Gränna-Museerna, Gränna, Sweden, provided photographs and allowed their reproduction; Ulla Curran read and commented on the final draft.

'The Visitor from a Far Country': Dr David Van Zwanenberg, whose article (cited in our references) needs to be the starting point for any reassessment of this outbreak of plague in Suffolk, talked to us and gave us the freedom of his files; Mrs Hewett, formerly librarian to Ipswich Hospital Medical Library, provided access to the Dr H. P. Sleigh collection of documents and other material in the library archives; and Ronald Blythe, Dr K. T. Brown and David Dymond read and commented on the final draft.

'The Walk to Eternity': the Mawson Institute for Antarctic Research, University of Adelaide, Australia, was especially co-operative in supplying photostats of relevant portions of Sir Douglas Mawson's diaries and in making a set of fine prints from the original glass plates and giving permission for us to use them.

We are grateful, too, for the existence of, and facilities

offered by, the following libraries, as well as for the unfailing helpfulness of their staff: the Barnes Medical Library, University of Birmingham, and its librarian, Mr S. R. Jenkins; the Library of the Wellcome Institute for the History of Medicine; and the London Library. And we wish to record our thanks to Churchill College in the University of Cambridge for allowing us to meet and work on its premises from time to time.

Both Greta Howell and Chloë Jowett read our drafts in various phases and made helpful suggestions for improvements. The ladies of Palmer Brown Office Services, Halesowen, handled the typing of many of the provisional drafts, while Jane Turner and Susan Ashdown looked after the typing of certain episodes in their intermediate stages. Vanessa Young then dealt with the final typing, working to a testing schedule that allowed us to honour a delivery date. We also wish to express our appreciation of the forbearance and encouragement of our editor, Eleo Gordon, throughout many months of writing.

West Midlands and   M. H.
Suffolk   P. F.
November 1984

Chapter 1

═══════════════════════════════════════

The Stranded Eagle

When the Swedish gunboat *Svenskund* set sail down the long sound from Gothenberg harbour, it carried on board a party of three explorers who were starting out on a remarkable quest. This was a second try. An attempt made the previous year had failed, but now, at six o'clock in the evening, on 18 May 1897, the explorers were full of confidence. Their objective was among the most elusive goals of nineteenth-century geographical ventures, to reach the North Pole, and they were proposing to do so by means of a mammoth balloon.

It is hard to read accounts of their setting out without being irresistibly reminded of the novels of Jules Verne. Like so many of that writer's fictional but prophetic enterprises, the expedition was founded on the most up-to-date advances in Victorian technology. Its very conception needed the practicalities of both science and engineering to be stretched far beyond the limits of experience. The explorers were equipped to continue to lead, as they travelled, the lives of nineteenth-century gentlemen. Their provisions list included almost everything imaginable, from woollen undershirts and drawers to theodolites and scientific almanacs, from sporting guns and bottles of excellent wine to carrier pigeons and a prefabricated boat. Their outer clothing was stout, sensible and decidedly tweedy.

The trio's bold undertaking fired the public imagination, and provoked in almost every European country controversy and debate. Pessimists predicted how birds would peck holes in the balloon, how the explorers would be shot by savages or suffocated by the attenuated atmosphere. One Austrian newspaper went so far as to brand the expedition's leader either fool or swindler, and even reputable scientists and explorers were divided in their opinions. In Britain, the Arctic explorers Admiral Markham and General Greely thought the plan ill-advised, but in France the project, after being debated by the Academy of Sciences, received qualified approval. At the Meteorological Institute in Berlin it was enthusiastically acclaimed, and in Sweden itself the expedition, backed by generous donations from King Oscar II as well as from Alfred Nobel, the inventor of dynamite and later founder of the Nobel Prize awards, became a focus for intense national pride. The explorers were being hailed as heroes even before their expedition was under way.

The leader of the expedition, whose concept it was and on whom much of the limelight would inevitably fall, was a 43-year-old scientist and engineer, Salomon August Andrée. Andrée already enjoyed a considerable reputation, not only as chief engineer to the Swedish Patent Office and founder of the Society of Swedish Inventors, but also as a passionate advocate of the hydrogen balloon, recommending it as a vehicle for scientific research as well as for geographical exploration.

The first of his fellow explorers for the flight was Nils Strindberg, a 25-year-old assistant from the physics department of the University of Stockholm who was also a distant relative of the playwright August Strindberg. He was doubly qualified for the expedition, being a highly talented amateur photographer as well as a scientist. The other companion was

Knut Fraenkel, a sturdily built, athletically inclined civil engineer in his late twenties. Inevitably Fraenkel was to find himself cast in the role of the practical man or brawn of the party, but both had taken care to obtain some actual experience in ballooning, Strindberg having made six ascents, Fraenkel seven.

Andrée himself was an experienced balloonist, having made a series of nine, extremely bold, single-handed ascents in his own balloon, travelling an accumulated distance of over 900 miles and achieving a total flying time of forty hours. His longest flight, which lasted ten and a half hours, had carried him 240 miles and included a crossing of the Baltic. His personal altitude record stood at 14,250 feet. During these flights he had recorded more than 400 scientific observations, studying everything from meteorology to aerial photography and even carrying a hand mirror so that he might check at various heights for changes in his complexion. He was earnest and sincere, if rather over self-important, and he believed devoutly in the benefits which technology held out for mankind. But if he was idealistic he was also ambitious. The flight to the North Pole was meant not only to demonstrate the practical importance of the hydrogen balloon and aeronautics, but also to consolidate his reputation on an international basis.

Every detail of Andrée's epic project was meticulously planned. The balloon, packed carefully away in the hold of the *Svenskund*, had been specially built for its task. Christened *Örnen* (the *Eagle*), it had been constructed in Paris under the close supervision of a Swedish engineer by the famous balloon-maker Henri Lachambre. From its original design it was enlarged by the insertion of extra panels above and below its equator so that it became slightly elliptical in outline with a diameter of nearly eighty feet. Fully inflated with hydrogen, it had a capacity of 170,000 cubic feet and was capable of lifting a weight of more than five tons. It was made from varnished Chinese silk: a single layer in the lower hemisphere, but reinforced to three layers in the upper hemisphere.

The whole balloon was enclosed in net made from Italian hemp soaked in acid-free Vaseline so it would not absorb moisture. At the lower pole of the balloon the net ended in a series of forty-eight ropes anchored to the carrying-ring from which the car or basket was to be suspended. Over the upper quarter of the balloon a further layer of varnished silk was fashioned into a *calotte* or cap which fitted outside the netting. This served the double purpose of preventing snow and ice from collecting in the interstices of the net while trapping a layer of air to provide thermal insulation against sudden changes in temperature which could alter the balloon's buoyancy. The standard practice of placing a valve at the apex of the balloon was abandoned in case it became frozen or obstructed by snow. Instead, two valves were provided at different heights on the overhanging flanks of the lower hemisphere. The mouth of the balloon was closed by a Gifford safety-valve which allowed any excessive pressure within the balloon to leak away.

The balloon-car which was to hang from the carrying-ring consisted of a circular wickerwork basket, five feet deep and six and a half feet in diameter. Roofed in and protected on every side by canvas, it also incorporated three cramped berths and was capable of storing considerable quantities of provisions. The roof of the balloon-car, protected by canvas and guarded by a rail, formed an observation platform from which the explorers could navigate. Extra equipment would be carried in various pockets and baskets lashed high in the rigging above the carrying-ring.

The *Örnen* had two novel features: it was equipped with trailing ropes and sails, all part of an ingenious system devised to regulate its flight. There were two sets of ropes which trailed below the balloon. First there were the three 'trailing-lines', each 1,100 feet long and weighing over five hundredweight, which were attached to the carrying-ring by a swivelling-block. Second there were eight shorter ballast ropes, each 230 feet long and weighing about a hundredweight.

It was intended that the balloon should journey at a low altitude to conserve lifting power. At greater heights, where the atmospheric pressure was less, the hydrogen in the balloon would expand and gas be lost by both leakage at the safety-valve and increased percolation through the Chinese silk. To keep the balloon floating at between 450 and 500 feet, approximately a third of each of the three long trailing-lines would rest on the surface of the sea or ice. Any rise in altitude would then, it was thought, automatically increase the load upon the balloon as more rope was lifted and carried. With the trailing-lines lifted clear of the surface, an additional five or six hundredweight would be added to the weight supported. Conversely, as the balloon sank, an increased weight of trailing-lines and ballast ropes would rest on the surface. In theory, the balloon could lose as much as eighteen and a half hundredweight of lifting power before the car actually touched down.

With considerable resourcefulness, this simple self-regulating altitude control had been adapted one stage further. It was obvious that the trailing-lines, by dragging on sea or ice, must impede progress. The balloon would travel rather more slowly than the wind pushing it along; air currents would be constantly sweeping past. Hence a sail placed obliquely in these currents must necessarily act as a rudder and steer the balloon to one side or the other. Experiments suggested that a balloon could be guided into travelling at an angle as sharp as 30° from the direct line of the wind direction. Three square sails, having a total area of 800 square feet, were therefore rigged on horizontal bamboo spars. The sails were fixed, but could be adjusted in their inclination to the wind simply by winching the whole balloon round on the swivelling-block which supported the trailing-lines.

Andrée had allowed his designs to be modified in only one detail. The three long trailing-lines were each interrupted at mid-point by the insertion of a screw connector similar to those used to join drain-rods. Should any single rope become tangled in an object on the ground, the balloon could now be freed simply by twisting the upper end of the trailing-line.

On 30 May the *Svenskund* reached Spitsbergen. The balloon's launch was to take place from Virgo Harbour, a sheltered site on the northern shore of Danes Island at Spitsbergen's north-western tip. Here, during the abortive attempt to launch the balloon the previous year, a special balloon house had been built so the balloon could wait for the essential southerly winds while protected from Arctic storms. Roughly circular in layout, with a diameter of ninety-five feet and walls over a hundred feet high, the balloon house was constructed so that the whole front half of the building could be dismantled to let the balloon float free.

For the second time, therefore, provisions and equipment were carried ashore, the hydrogen apparatus erected, the balloon installed, examined and inflated. By 1 July, preparations were complete. Everything hung on the elements. In 1896, the expedition had waited vainly for a suitable wind. Now, as if to jest at their presumptions, the weather maintained a resolute calm for days on end. At last, on 11 July, in the early hours of the morning, cats-paws were seen disturbing the surface of the water in the anchorage. A wind sprang up at last. As the morning brightened, the wind swung round to the north, blowing in gusts as strong as ten or twenty miles an hour. Amid a sudden turmoil of hasty, last-minute preparations, however, Andrée hesitated over taking the decision to fly. When it came to it there seemed to be a sudden loss of nerve among the explorers. Asked for his opinion on whether to launch, Fraenkel answered evasively at first, before declaring they should start. Strindberg said that he felt they ought to attempt it. Andrée, still hesitating, finally committed himself with the words: 'My comrades insist on starting, and as I have no fully valid reasons against it, I shall agree to it, although with some reluctance.'

The front of the balloon house was dismantled, the balloon allowed to rise a few feet on its moorings, the car attached to the carrying-ring. Final provisions were brought from the ship, the instruments checked and the balloonists helped aboard. At 1.46 p.m., amid a flurry of goodwill messages and the thin cheers of the shore working party, the three anchoring ropes were cut and the balloon surged strongly from its moorings.

Almost immediately there was pandemonium. With a single, strong bound the balloon lifted clear of the balloon house and set out across the bay, then hung for a moment before sinking at a catastrophic speed. With frantic haste the travellers jettisoned ballast. For a moment the car touched the surface of the water, dragged forward and began to dip. Then, with a sharp lurch, the balloon lifted and began to climb, the trailing ballast-lines leaving wide furrows across the waters of Virgo Harbour. In the ensuing turmoil, a workman shouted out that the three long drag-lines had separated from the balloon and been left behind. Laid out, as they were, along the beach ahead of the balloon, it seemed they had somehow

become twisted and unscrewed themselves at the metal
connections. All the elaborate plans to guide-rope the balloon,
stabilize its height and control its direction were thus frustrated before the flight was properly begun.

For thirty-five minutes the observers on the shore watched
as the *Örnen* became a small spot low in the sky and moving
steadily northwards. Slowly it rose and cleared a distant
headland before being lost in a haze of fine mist and cloud.

Four days later the skipper of a Norwegian sealer, the *Alken*,
was summoned on deck in the early hours of the morning
after a 'peculiar bird' settled on the peak of the ship. It had
flown from the south, pursued by two ivory gulls. The skipper
thought the bird looked something like a ptarmigan, climbed
the rigging and shot it. Unfortunately the bird fell into the
sea. Later that day, meeting another sealer, the story was
recounted and, although neither skipper knew whether the
balloon was yet launched, it was suggested the bird might
have been one of Andrée's carrier-pigeons. The *Alken*
returned to the region where the bird had been shot, lowered
two boats and, surprisingly enough, managed to find the
bird's body. Strapped to its central tail feather was a small
metal dispatch cylinder which contained the briefest of
messages:

From Andrée's Polar Expedition to
        Aftonbladet, Stockholm.
13th July
12.30 midday, Lat. 82° 2' Long. 15° 5' E. good
speed to E. 10° south. All well on
board. This is the third pigeon-post.
                    Andrée

If estimates of position could be trusted, the expedition
must therefore have travelled 175 miles, a quarter of the

distance to the Pole, during the first forty-eight hours of flight. The expedition carried thirty-six pigeons, but none of the others ever reappeared.

On 3 November, four months after the launching, a relief expedition sailed from Tromsö to investigate reports of mysterious calls having been heard from Spitsbergen and of the balloon being seen floating in the sea. Experienced Arctic travellers inclined to the view that the cries would be those of sea birds and the object reported as a balloon probably a dead whale. The most eminent authorities on the Arctic considered it extremely unlikely that Andrée's expedition was still anywhere in the vicinity of Spitsbergen. It was thought more probable that he could have made a landfall somewhere on the north coasts of America or Asia, and that, after over-wintering, he would make his way back in the spring. More forebodingly, however, they felt that if he had come down on the ice anywhere between 83° north and the Pole it would be practically impossible for him to extract himself. On the 21st the relief expedition returned empty-handed.

Then, on 4 May 1899, almost two years after the *Örnen* set out, a damaged marker buoy was found lying on the beach of a fjord on the northern coast of Iceland. The expedition had carried twelve such buoys, each made of cork and weighing about four and a half pounds. The buoys were to be used as dispatch boxes. Inside the watertight compartment of the damaged buoy, on quite a large sheet of paper, was the briefest of messages:

This buoy has been thrown from Andrée's balloon at 10 h. 55 m. GMT in about 82° latitude and 25° long, E. fr. Gr.[eenwich] We are floating at a height of 600 metres [1,950 feet].

All well.

Andrée Strindberg Fraenkel

Four months later Andrée's polar buoy, a rather larger buoy which he had intended dropping at the Pole or the most northerly point they managed to reach, was picked up on the beach of King Charles Land to the north-east of Spitsbergen. Its watertight message compartment was empty.

One further buoy turned up on the north-west tip of Norway on 27 August 1900. It contained the longest dispatch of all:

Buoy No. 4 The first
thrown out
on the 11th July, 10 p.m. G.M.T.

Our journey has hitherto gone well. We are still moving on at a height of 250 m. [830 feet] in a direction which was at first N. 10° E. declination, but later N. 45° E. declination. Four carrier-pigeons were sent off at 5 h. 40 p.m. Greenw. time. They flew westerly. We are now in over the ice, which is much broken up in all directions. Weather magnificent. In best of humours.

Andrée Strindberg Fraenkel

Above the clouds since 7.45 G.M.T.

In the years that followed three or four other buoys were cast up on lonely beaches around the edge of the Arctic Circle. None, however, contained any words or clues. The Arctic drew an impenetrable veil over Andrée's fate.

It was in 1930 that a Norwegian sealer, the *Bratvaag*, sailed for Franz Josef Land, carrying a party of scientists on what was planned as a combined hunting and research expedition. They were fortunate with the weather. The Arctic summer that year was exceptionally mild, the ice-fields had retreated to the north and it was now possible to reach and land on several small islands which ice and heavy swell normally made inaccessible. Among several islands visited by the *Bratvaag* was White Island, a barren outcrop of ice-capped rock, seventeen miles long and eight to ten miles broad, which lay thirty miles off the mainland of the easternmost portion of the Spitsbergen archipelago.

For twenty-four hours shore parties hunted for walrus and conducted a series of scientific studies. Then, on 6 August, two young seamen, pausing to search for fresh water, stumbled across the remnants of a camp. There were sledges as well as a boat half-submerged in the ice at the foot of a low outcrop of broken rock. One of the first objects to be freed from the ice and lifted from the interior of the boat was a brass boat-hook engraved: 'Andrée's pol. exp. 1896'. A careful search by the shore parties revealed the outlines of a tent, provisions, guns and ammunition, a vast and bewildering array of scientific equipment, even books and mathematical tables. Among the objects finally recovered were the personal journals of the explorers and the expedition's camera and undeveloped films. At last, from the journals and photographs developed from the films, it became possible to reconstruct the journey that had been accomplished.

The North Pole lay a little more than 700 miles distant from the balloon house on Danes Island. With a direct flight at an average speed, a balloon could theoretically accomplish such a journey in about thirty hours. Andrée, Strindberg and Fraenkel, as they clutched frantically for handholds on the guard-rail and rigging when the balloon flopped precipitously into the waters of the harbour at the outset, must have realized in their hearts that this aim was now impossible. Even as the *Örnen* staggered up into the freshening wind, shorn of its long trailing-lines and with 450 pounds of precious ballast already jettisoned, Fraenkel was forced to clamber precariously into the upper rigging to take in the sails, the unbalanced pull of the remaining heavy ballast ropes having swung the balloon round so that the sails in fact hampered and depressed its flight.

Nevertheless they were sweeping towards the north-east at a steady twenty miles an hour, lifting gradually from the grey sea to pass above the frozen headland of Vogelsang. To the watchers on the shore, it seemed that the balloon disappeared into a fine mist. The aeronauts, however, found themselves entering a fog, and under its cold, sunless influence the *Örnen* seemed to lose buoyancy and sink. Within minutes, the truncated drag-lines were trailing on the surface of the water. For a while the balloon floated in eerie silence, but then, as it broke free from the mist, buoyancy suddenly returned and it climbed steadily towards a blue sky and an altitude of nearly 2,000 feet. Already the balloonists could hear the low whine of gas escaping from the Gifford safety-valve. It became clear that the giant balloon was unexpectedly and perhaps disastrously sensitive to the slightest change in temperature. The difference between sunshine and shadow meant the difference between rising and falling.

Yet, suspended high in the bright sunlight, the *Örnen* swept steadily north-east, drifting above a turquoise sea pockmarked by white slabs of floating ice. On the observation platform the balloonists struggled to draw up the remnants of the trailing-lines, splicing one to another to form a single makeshift drag-line of reasonable length. By late afternoon they were crossing the first of the pack-ice – drifting ice-floes separated from one another by leads of clear water. Far below them a solitary seagull accompanied their progress.

During the early evening the air beneath thickened imperceptibly into a mist, and by 7 p.m. they were moving slowly through a silent world of pale sunlight above a dark sea of cloud. They took turns to sleep. All day they had listened to the whine of gas escaping from the safety-valve, and now those on watch found it necessary to drop ballast again and again as the balloon sunk ominously towards the cold mists below. At one o'clock in the morning the wind failed, and for almost two hours they hung motionless in the twilit world of an Arctic summer night. At last the merest breath of cold air came whispering from the east. The wind had shifted. As day advanced and the breeze freshened into a strong wind, they were swept steadily westward, sinking down through a dripping grey mist to as close to surface level as sixty-five feet. Crumpled ice-fields slipped beneath them, not white as they had expected, but coloured with a faded yellowish tint that exactly matched the fur of the polar bear.

The mist seemed to cling about the balloon, dripping from the rigging and weighing them down so that they barely cleared the ice. In mid-afternoon the balloon-car twice grounded heavily before sluggishly lifting again into the mist. At ever more frequent intervals they jettisoned ballast and various items of equipment, and at 4.15 p.m., in what must have been a painful acknowledgement of the expedition's failure, discarded the polar buoy itself. By now the balloon was travelling at a leisurely five miles an hour, and they sank even lower until the balloon-car struck the ice over and over again, dragging and bumping in slow ungainly hops which carried it 150 yards at a time. For more than six hours the grinding, shuddering progress continued. Then, at ten o'clock at night, it suddenly ceased. The trailing line had caught under a block of ice; the balloon was tethered. For almost thirteen hours it remained anchored, twisting, eddying, rising and falling restlessly on the end of its guide-rope. Strindberg and Fraenkel seized the chance to sleep. Andrée, keeping watch alone, confided his thoughts to his diary:

Although we could have thrown out ballast and although the wind might, perhaps, carry us to Greenland, we determined to be content with standing still. We have been obliged to throw out very much ballast today and have not had any sleep nor been allowed any rest from the repeated bumpings, and we probably could not have stood it much longer. All three of us must have a rest . . .

It is not a little strange to be floating here above the Polar Sea. To be the first that have floated here in a balloon. How soon, I wonder, shall we have successors? Shall we be thought mad or will our example be followed? I cannot deny but that all three of us are dominated by a feeling of pride. We think we can well face death, having done what we have done. Is not the whole, perhaps, the expression of an extremely strong sense of individuality which cannot bear the thought of living and dying like a man in the ranks, forgotten by coming generations? Is this ambition?

The next day seemed brighter than any of them had dared to hope. The sun broke through the haze, the wind was again blowing steadily towards the north-east and the balloon regained its buoyancy. At ten o'clock it broke free of its own accord and rose again confidently. For a while the journey proceeded steadily and they had hopes of a high-altitude flight, but by midday the sun was lost behind a thickening haze. There was a fresh coldness in the air. Before long the water dripping from the rigging and envelope froze into layers of brittle ice. By 10.30 that night the balloon-car was again crashing into the ice, staggering and rebounding from hummock to hummock. The night hours passed in a nerve-racking ordeal of violent shocks. At seven the next morning Andrée finally accepted defeat, opened the valves to release the hydrogen and brought the balloon down in a proficient landing that threw the balloon-car on its side but injured none of the balloonists and damaged none of their vital equipment.

Inexplicably it was an hour and a half before the explorers actually stepped from the balloon. They then set about establishing a camp and spent several days unloading, packing the sledges, assembling and testing the canvas boat and checking provisions. They were about 200 miles from the nearest land, but repeated checks on their position suggested that the two vast ice-floes on which they had landed were drifting south-south-west at between four and five miles a day.

On 22 July they broke camp, having chosen to attempt a long haul to the south and safety rather than wait passively to see where the slow drift of the great ice-field would carry them. They had a choice of two destinations: the Spitsbergen archipelago to the south-west or Franz Josef Land to the south-east. It was 192 miles to land adjacent to north-east Spitsbergen and 216 miles to Franz Josef Land. A small depot of provisions had been established for them at Seven Islands off Spitsbergen, and a larger depot at Cape Flora in Franz Josef Land. They chose Franz Josef Land. Nansen had already proved it possible to survive an Arctic winter sheltering there, and it offered the added attraction that much of the route lay through regions which were largely unexplored. They were tragically unaware of how the great westward sweep of the Arctic currents must inevitably frustrate any attempt to march east across the drifting ice.

The journey on which they now embarked was to take them almost three months. They were attempting to move more than half a ton of provisions and equipment, including an unwieldy boat, 200 miles across an infinitely fragmented terrain. Even on their best days they never achieved an advance of more than a few miles. It took them almost two weeks of struggle to realize that the prospect of reaching Franz Josef Land was negligible. Hastily they turned towards the south-west. For a further six weeks they struggled desperately in the direction of Seven Islands, only to find any hard-won progress repeatedly stolen away by the imperceptible drift of the immense ice-field. At last, the Arctic winter almost upon them, they abandoned their march and prepared to weather it out on the open pack-ice, allowing the Arctic currents to carry them where they would.

From the beginning their march was a protracted ordeal of muscular effort and personal suffering. Their sledges were grossly overloaded, each one carrying between 390 and 420 pounds in weight. They could only move a sledge by combined effort. Together they manhandled each sledge in turn a few hundred yards before returning for the next. At the outset it was clear that the loads would have to be reduced, and even by the second day of the journey the sledges were beginning to break up under the strain. Yet it was two further days before any firm decision was taken to abandon items of stores and equipment and reduce the load on each sledge by over 100 pounds. They were casting aside a considerable portion of their food supply, retaining enough for only forty-five days. Before resuming their journey, however, they indulged in the largest meal possible, washing it all down with a bottle of no doubt adequately chilled champagne.

If they were to survive they were going to have to rely on their skill as hunters. Fortunately, polar bears seemed to be attracted to their camp, and they quickly developed a certain rough expertise in killing them. In the tradition of the successful Victorian shooting party, they photographed each other standing triumphantly beside their huge trophies. Altogether they killed about a dozen polar bears; on two separate occasions they even succeeded in killing a she-bear and two cubs within a few moments. One of the bears that Andrée killed, an elderly he-bear, was described by his companions as 'the oldest bear in the polar regions', 'an escaped menagerie bear', 'as tough as leather galoshes', but as a rule they found the meat palatable. They discarded the liver and thought fried bear heart was slightly bitter. The tongue, kidneys and brain, on the other hand, as well as fillets cut from the ribs, were especially acceptable. It helped to immerse the carcass in sea-water brine for a while, or to wait until the meat was some days old. Bear ham several days old was considered a gourmet's treat.

They found that carrying their day's meat supply close to the body prevented it from freezing. Their communal reindeer-hide sleeping-sack was moulting and Andrée noted drily: '*A little* reindeer-hair in the food is recommended for while taking it out one is prevented from eating too quickly and greedily.' They even took to eating the bear meat uncooked. An entry in Andrée's diary for 21 August 1897 reads: 'This evening on my proposal we tasted what raw meat was like. Raw bear with salt tastes like oysters and we hardly wanted to fry it. Raw brain is also very good and the bear's meat was easily eaten raw.' They even evolved a recipe for 'blood pancakes', mixing oatmeal with the blood and frying it in butter. The result was considered 'quite excellent'. Although they were daily consuming up to two and a half pounds of bear meat apiece, they still held considerable stores of European foods, including bread, biscuits, butter, sugar, sardines, coffee and canned milk.

Progress across the ice-fields continued to be obstructed by innumerable obstacles, and inevitably they came to rely heavily upon Fraenkel's superior physique. Their sledges had to be dragged or lifted over huge blocks of ice and narrow pressure ridges. In places the corroded surface of the ice was combined with snow to produce layers of finely powdered 'sugar-snow' in which their feet slipped but the sledge runners stuck tight as glue. They picked their way between pools and canals of melted fresh water, but often discovered them only by crashing through thin layers of newly formed ice on their surface. Three or four times each day their route was blocked by open leads where the sea had formed wide channels between ice-floes. Sometimes they launched the boat; more often they managed to improvise a bridge or ferry supplies on a convenient raft of drifting ice.

Periodic illness had also begun to hamper their journey even in the early stages. Within a week of their trek beginning Fraenkel was showing early symptoms of snow-blindness. The cold seemed to penetrate their nostrils and they found themselves with persistent catarrh and running noses. Before long Fraenkel was disturbing the others' sleep as he clambered from the communal sleeping-sack to cope with attacks of diarrhoea.

The sheer effort of the unanticipated and unaccustomed exercise had a sapping effect on their spirits and strength. On 9 August Andrée noted in his diary: 'F. has diarrhoea for 2nd time and there does not seem much left of his moral strength . . . We were tired out and F. was ill. I gave him opium for the diarrhoea.' And, on the following day: 'We have gone into our tent after only 7 hours' march but it was so dreadfully fatiguing . . . F.'s stomach pains are now over.'

For a while things went rather more smoothly, but, on 15 August, Strindberg and Andrée both fell victims to diarrhoea. Nils Strindberg already had a cut hand swathed in bandages as well as a boil on his upper lip. Then, on the 22nd, Fraenkel suffered what was probably an injury to his knee cartilage. Andrée recorded: 'I massaged F.'s foot. He had been pulling so that his knee went out of joint but it slipped in again but he had no bad effects of it.' Nils Strindberg developed a painful toe, though there was no obvious cause. It was a catalogue of minor upsets, except that the circumstances made every minor upset a serious matter.

Within forty-eight hours they were again in trouble. Indeed, Tuesday, 24 August, seemed to mark the start of a particularly bad spell of ill-health for the party. Knut Fraenkel was dogged for several days by recurrent diarrhoea, severe stomach pains and episodes of cramp which Andrée tried to relieve by massage. He treated Nils Strindberg's painful toe by rubbing boot grease inside the sock, but the discomfort persisted. The next day Andrée himself was overcome by diarrhoea. On 27 August he noted: 'F. has again had very bad diarrhoea and has got opium. I have had diarrhoea too today but I imagine I am well again now without any medicine.' On the 28th he wrote somewhat bitterly: 'F. is bad again. Yesterday he got an opium tablet against diarrhoea and this evening he has got a morphine tablet against the pains in his stomach we shall see if he can become a man again [*sic*].'

At midnight on Tuesday, 31 August, the sun touched the horizon for the first time and for a few minutes it seemed to Andrée, now under the influence of both an opium and a morphine tablet, that the snow and ice had turned into a sea of fire. It was a warning that the Arctic summer was almost over, but the explorers, overcome with exhaustion, spent the following day quietly resting and repairing equipment. Poor Andrée, having crept from the tent during the night because of his diarrhoea, had discovered himself being inspected by an open-mouthed bear.

Nils Strindberg's birthday fell on 4 September, and Andrée awoke him to give him letters from his sweetheart and relatives. Andrée, who once confessed to being afraid to marry because he would never dare to submit to the powerful

emotions thus released, nevertheless took considerable pleasure in Strindberg's joy. He had been carrying the letters
since they left Sweden.

The leads between the ice-floes were by now wider and
more frequent, the explorers therefore suspecting that they
were moving close to the edge of the pack-ice. On 5 September
they launched their boat and were able to row for six hours
without landing. By 9 September both Andrée and Fraenkel
had recovered from their diarrhoea. Fraenkel's foot, however,
was still causing trouble, a large pus-blister needing to be
opened. His foot became so bad that he could no longer pull
his sledge, managing only to push it from behind, his
companions taking turns with coming back to help him. One
of Strindberg's feet was also troublesome.

Throughout 12 and 13 September their journey was interrupted by a violent storm which forced them to lie up in their
tents. During these two days they finally resigned themselves
to wintering on the pack-ice. They were encamped on an ice-
floe, eighty yards wide and over a hundred yards long, their
observations revealing that it was being swept due south into
the gap between Spitsbergen and Franz Josef Land at a rate
of almost thirty miles a day. Animal life was becoming more
plentiful and they managed to kill seals for food, as well as
various birds.

On 15 September they sighted land: a long low island, the
surface of which was almost completely concealed beneath a
glacier. They identified it correctly as White Island and were
greatly encouraged to find their ice-floe carrying them rapidly
towards it. On 18 September, in high spirits and still sailing
serenely past the ice cliffs of White Island, they celebrated. It
was the twenty-fifth anniversary of the ascension of their
patron, Oscar II, to the Swedish throne. They raised the
Swedish flag and finished the day with a ceremonial dinner

which included a 65-year-old bottle of vintage port. Strind-berg recorded their menu:

Banquet 18 Sept. 97
on an ice-floe immediately east of [White Island]

Seal steak and ivory gull fried in butter and seal-blubber, seal liver, - brain and kidneys. Butter and Schumacher bread.
Wine.
Chocolate and Mellin's-food flour with Albert biscuits and butter.
Gâteau aux raisin.
Raspberry syrup sauce.
Port-wine 1834 Antonio de Ferrara given by the King.
Toast by Andrée for the King with royal Hurrah:
The national anthem in unison.
Biscuits, butter, cheese.
A glass of wine.
Festive feeling . . .

In the succeeding days they made no attempt to land, allowing the steady drift of wind and currents to sweep them down the island's eastern coast before swinging them round south until they were almost at its western point. They were living in tolerable comfort in the hut of frozen snow blocks which Strindberg built as a 'permanent' base on the ice, and had accumulated enough meat to see them through the winter.

On the morning of 2 October they were awoken at five-thirty by a violent shock as the ice-floe split into smaller segments. One fissure, which passed immediately beneath the walls of the hut, brought water rushing into their sleeping quarters. Their ice-raft was now only eighty feet wide, and three days later they reluctantly abandoned it and carried equipment and provisions safely across a series of floes to the shore. At last they stood on solid ground.

Their diaries now contained scraps of information about setting up camp, reconnoitring, shifting camp a little further inland. The last entry in Andrée's journal was dated 8 October. Reconstructed from a badly damaged fragment it reads:

During the 8th the weather was bad and we had to keep to the tent all day. Still we fetched enough driftwood so we could lay the beams for the roof of our house. It feels fine to be able to sleep on fast land as a contrast with the drifting ice out upon the ocean, where we constantly heard the cracking, grinding and din. We shall have to gather driftwood and bones of whales, and we shall have to do some moving around when the weather permits.

The exposed film in the camera had deteriorated by the time it was found, but eventually about sixteen quite acceptable prints were salvaged. They showed views from the balloon, the stranded balloon on the ice and various incidents from the journey across the pack-ice. There were no pictures from White Island.

Strindberg's almanac had one last note scribbled in the margin on 17 October. It was only brief: 'home: 7.5 o'cl a.m.' Unlike his preceding pencilled notes, this one was written in ink.

The rest was silence.

It was going to take two expeditions to uncover and retrieve all the artefacts from the camp on White Island, the party from the *Bratvaag* being followed only a month later by a second expedition aboard the sealer *Isbjörn*, chartered especially by a newspaper syndicate.

The camp, the *Bratvaag* group found, had been established about 250 yards from the shore, directly against a low outcrop of rock. This ridge, a low escarpment of gravel and boulder, ran almost due east and west, rising in three gradual steps to a height of perhaps sixteen or twenty feet. The camp lay at its foot, facing out to sea and the north-west. The space where the tent once stood was a large rectangular area delineated by a regular pattern of driftwood logs and the bones of a whale evidently used to anchor down the canvas edges. The tent had in fact been pitched so that the lower ridge of boulders virtually formed a rear wall to the living accommodation.

Not far to the west of the tent area lay two sledges. One of these, probably Andrée's, had evidently been used to carry the tent with its accessories, for it stood empty and unloaded. The second was Fraenkel's. This lay almost concealed beneath the canvas boat which had been pushed on top of it. The boat was full to the brim with neatly packed layers of stores and equipment. Strindberg's sledge stood some thirty feet further off, where it was eventually found by the *Isbjörn* party. Close by was a large section of balloon cloth which seemed to have been used as a tarpaulin and a scattered collection of snow-shoes, scientific instruments, clothing and provision baskets. Knut Stubbendorff, who led the *Isbjörn* expedition, concluded that this part of the camp had been used as a material depot. On the eastern side of the tent area was heaped a considerable stack of salvaged driftwood.

The most important, disturbing and, indeed, puzzling discoveries made by the two ships' parties, however, were the three explorers' remains. The first body to be found gave the impression of lying almost naturally against the slightly sloping rock wall within the tent. It was still almost hidden by the drifts of snow and ice, the legs clad in trousers and Lapp boots, although the top half of the body had been drastically disturbed. The head and whole upper portion were missing, while the bones of a pelvis were found some sixty yards away. It was assumed that polar bears must have ravaged the corpse when ransacking the camp, but from markings on the back of a waistcoat associated with these bones it became clear that the body was Andrée's. Beside him on the rocks, as though ready for immediate use, lay a gun and the primus cooking stove.

A second body was found about thirty-five yards from the tent in a typical Arctic grave. It had been laid in a deep cleft between the rocks and covered by a mound of heavy boulders. Evidently the marauding bears managed to break into even this simple tomb, and the presence of the body was given away not only by the pair of Lapp boots which protruded from among the disturbed stones but also by a bare skull which lay grinning next to the rocks. Initials carefully stitched into the clothing showed that here were the remains of Nils Strindberg.

The collected human remnants were enclosed in a specially constructed wooden chest with two compartments which was to be carried on the after-deck. The *Bratvaag* then resumed her voyage to Franz Josef Land, everything which could be hewn free from the ice having been gathered up and put aboard. Two days later the *Bratvaag* met up with a homeward-bound sealer, and entrusted a message announcing the discovery of the Andrée campsite to the skipper. By the time the message was delivered in Tromsö, the sealer's skipper was prepared to swear he had seen Andrée's body aboard the *Bratvaag*, frozen intact in clear ice so that even the features could be recognized.

By the time the *Isbjörn* arrived, the continuing summer thaw allowed further objects to be found, and now Fraenkel's body was discovered. It was within the tent area, only three or four feet from where Andrée had lain. Andrée's skull as well as bones from his arm and upper skeleton were also found. When the *Isbjörn* returned to Tromsö, Andrée's coffin was brought from where it lay in state before the cathedral altar so that his various fragments could be reunited.

The two expeditions eventually recovered almost a quarter of a ton of stores and equipment. During their slow journey across the ice-pack the explorers kept meticulous inventories, and practically every item mentioned in them was identified, along with quite a few objects not included in the lists. There were, on the other hand, no hints whatsoever to account for the fate which had overtaken Andrée and his two companions.

Their achievements were undeniable. They had made an epic flight, remaining airborne for longer than any previous balloonists. As the first to fly above the Arctic ice-cap, they had travelled nearly 500 miles in sixty-five hours, even though their flight had advanced them only 240 miles in a straight line. They had accomplished a heroic march southwards from the 83rd parallel, across a drifting, unstable ice-field to reach the safety of a camp situated on the terra firma of White Island, and once there knew precisely where they were: within thirty miles of success and safety. On clear days they could even have seen the island of Storön, like a huge stepping-stone eighteen miles to the west, knowing that a mere nine miles beyond it lay North-East Land, part of the mainland of the Spitsbergen archipelago with its abundance of Arctic wildlife to stock their larder and occasional visits from passing sealers holding out a fair chance of rescue.

With success so nearly within their grasp why did the trio therefore perish? Their unexpected and apparently successive deaths have posed an enigma fit to puzzle the minds of fiction's great detectives, although many of the suggestions advanced can be discounted at once. They did not, for instance, die of starvation. Despite the ravages of the polar bears, some European food remained thirty-three years later, including such useful items as unopened tins of preserves and coffee. Steaks of meat cut from the back and ribs of a polar bear were packed in the boat. There were also two complete bear skins beside the tent as well as a pile of discarded bones from other bears and two seals, and the wings of at least a dozen ivory gulls. Uneaten food was even found on a plate and in a cooking pan within the actual tent area.

They could still hunt. All three of the party's guns were found, two in the boat, the third beside Andrée's body. There was plenty of ammunition. More bullets and shot cartridges were stocked on White Island than Nansen and Johansen carried to support themselves in the Arctic over at least two years during the *Fram* expedition of 1893–5.

The explanation arrived at by an official commission appointed to inquire into the White Island remains was that the explorers succumbed to cold, dying in their sleep from hypothermia. This theory was based almost entirely on comments made about the quality of the explorers' clothing by Professor Lithberg, a member of the committee:

One of the participators in the *Isbjörn* expedition expressed himself astonished at the unsuitability of the clothing for polar travelling. Among the articles he mentioned as being little suited to the purpose were the knitted gloves, the thin shirts of striped cotton, the thin woollen jerseys and short socks . . . Another man on board the *Isbjörn* gave it as his opinion that the members of the expedition had frozen to death. They did not have enough clothing and were badly equipped. They had nothing but rubbishy clothes and socks.

Several counter-arguments exist to this opinion, however, at least one Arctic explorer having discounted it on the grounds that it is air trapped between layers of clothing which gives insulation and warmth and that three or four layers of quite thin clothing can provide adequate protection. Rather than not having enough clothes, it was pointed out, the explorers were over-supplied, carrying a greater store of clothing than probably any Arctic expedition before them. Apart from the full and ample suits found on the three bodies, nineteen items of coats, shirts and jackets as well as sixty-three pairs of garments for legs, hands and feet and twenty-eight other articles of miscellaneous clothing were recovered.

It also seems strange that, if the explorers were suffering from cold, Andrée and Fraenkel were not found inside the communal sleeping-bag where they might have shared the warmth from one another's bodies. There was nothing to suggest that the bear skins had been used as blankets.

Yet the strongest argument against any theory of hypothermia lay in their fuel supply. When it was found beside Andrée's body, the primus stove was still in working order and three quarters full of paraffin. Later, when tested in Stockholm, it was found to be capable of boiling a litre of water in six minutes. There was a year's supply of matches and enough paraffin for at least a month. There was their stockpile of driftwood for burning and large quantities of blubber which could be used in 'fat-lamps'.

Nevertheless hypothermia remained the official explanation, although Vilhjalmur Stefansson, the Canadian-born Arctic explorer, using the same description of the camp as that available to the official committee, arrived at a different conclusion. His analysis began with the fact that Strindberg must have died first, his body having been buried in the simple Arctic grave. Stefansson therefore considered seven possible causes for Strindberg's death: an accidental gunshot wound, attack by a bear, suicide, murder by one of his companions, perhaps in a fit of insanity, drowning, food

poisoning and finally some such coincidental illness as
appendicitis or peritonitis.

Certain of these possibilities could be eliminated at once
on the grounds of circumstantial evidence. Both accidental
gunshot wound and attack by a bear could be dismissed since
there was no evidence of an appropriate injury to the skull or
skeleton while the suit of clothes in which Strindberg was
buried was neither torn nor pierced. Suicide could be discarded with confidence, Strindberg having maintained a
patient equanimity throughout the journey, the entries in his
journal being optimistic. Moreover, and most obviously, he
was now close not only to success and fame but to reunion
with his sweetheart. Murder by one of his companions even
in a fit of insanity was rejected for similar reasons: no damage
was done either to Strindberg's bones or his suit. In any case,
the journals portray a happy relationship between the explorers on the whole and their stresses must have been considerably less once their safety seemed assured.

Food poisoning was also ruled out by Stefansson. He noted
approvingly how they discarded the livers of the bears they
killed and attributed the explorers' digestive upsets to the
fact that they ate only lean meat. These symptoms seem to
have subsided once animal fat, in the form of 'blood-pan-
cakes', was included in their diet. He was confident that no
illness could be traced to the European food.

Thus only two possibilities remained among Stefansson's
theories: drowning or a serious illness. While feeling unable
to reach a definite conclusion, he preferred the theory of
drowning. He drew a picture of Strindberg in the excitement
of the chase, following a polar bear or seal on to the sea-ice
and falling through into the icy water. The scattered objects
which surrounded Strindberg's sledge leant support to the
idea. These he interpreted not as evidence of a material depot

but as an indication of Andrée and Fraenkel having torn from the sledge such items as a ladder to spread their weight over the thin ice and help them reach the spot where Strindberg fell through.

There remained two serious difficulties with this hypothesis. First, the sledge must afterwards have been carefully returned to the middle of the scattered circle of objects. Second, Strindberg's gun as well as Fraenkel's was found packed away in the boat while Andrée's lay beside his body.

For the deaths of Andrée and Fraenkel within the tent Stefansson put forward an intriguing theory. Besides being ingenious it had the advantage of accounting for why neither explorer made in his journal any record of a great misfortune befalling them. Noting the primus stove at Andrée's side, Stefansson suggested that both men died simultaneously from carbon monoxide poisoning caused by fumes from burning the primus in a confined space. To reinforce this idea, he speculated on how the tent could have become airtight as heavy snow drifted over it where it stood at the foot of its rock escarpment. He imagined the accident as having happened within hours of Strindberg's death.

For many years carbon monoxide poisoning was seen as the most likely explanation for the tragedy, even though certain difficulties remained unresolved. The tent, for instance, was no ordinary tent. Designed by Andrée, it was constructed from the lightest possible material: a single layer of balloon silk. The silk of the floor, varnished three times, had been stitched directly to the silk of the walls, varnished only once, and by the time the party reached White Island these layers of varnish must have been badly damaged. Then, instead of the usual 'bag-like' entrance to an Arctic tent which can be sealed by a 'purse-string' cord, this one was equipped only with door flaps. It was the unenviable fate of Andrée's tent to be castigated, on the one hand, by the official committee, who regarded it as flimsy, insubstantial and affording little protection, and on the other by Stefansson, who held it to be airtight and responsible for suffocating its owners.

There is, however, one weighty witness against the theory of carbon monoxide poisoning: the primus stove itself. It was in perfect working order when recovered, nearly full of paraffin and with its air-pressure valve closed. Had the explorers been overcome by the fumes and died with the stove working, it should have continued to burn until the fuel reservoir was empty. Alternatively, had the explorers become aware of their danger and struggled to extinguish the primus during their last few seconds of life, the air-pressure valve should have been open, releasing the pressure. Perhaps a strong draught then blew out the flame after the explorers had died, but that would indicate a degree of ventilation in which dangerous concentrations of fumes could hardly have accumulated.

The combination of a nearly full paraffin tank and a closed air valve was only to be explained in two ways: either the primus stove was not in use at all; or it had been lit in a sealed atmosphere so airtight that, within minutes of lighting it, the explorers died without warning, the flame of the stove being extinguished shortly afterwards by lack of oxygen. It seemed a rather far-fetched sequence of events in a tent of thin silk with an entrance closed only by flaps, even assuming that the tent had been freshly blanketed and sealed by falls of snow.

Despite its contradictions, Stefansson's theory of carbon monoxide poisoning continued to hold the field as the most likely explanation. Moreover, his careful consideration of the possible causes of Strindberg's death was quite convincing. Even if death by drowning was discounted, the suggestion remained that Strindberg maybe fell foul of a sudden, catastrophic illness.

Only in 1950 was another aspect of Stefansson's arguments looked at critically: the possibility of food poisoning. A Danish parasitologist, Dr Ernst Adam Tryde, after reading copies of the expedition's diaries, wondered whether the symptoms described might not be those of the disease trichinosis or trichinellosis, sometimes caused by eating meat which is contaminated by the larvae of a very small roundworm, *Trichinella spiralis* or *natira*. If such meat is inadequately cooked, the tiny larvae embedded in it survive to enter the victim's stomach and gut. Here they are released by the digestive process and anchor themselves to the mucosal lining of the intestine.

Within forty-eight hours the larvae mature into adult worms, the male worm then fertilizing the female before dying. The female burrows deep into the intestinal wall and within a week begins to give birth. Between 1,000 and 1,500 baby worms will be produced by one parent during the next four to six weeks, and, deposited in the intestinal mucosa, enter the lymphatic channels and eventually reach the bloodstream, which carries them to all parts of the body. Heart muscle and brain tissue may be damaged, injury to the heart occurring in direct proportion to the number of larvae that get into its flow of blood. Only in the voluntary or controlled muscles, however, can the young worms develop. Here they destroy the muscle fibrils and make the muscles sore and inflamed as they grow to a length of about a millimetre. Within a month they will be encapsulated in cysts.

Trichinosis is difficult to diagnose, its symptoms being extremely varied. The most consistent are probably the severe digestive disturbances which begin one to four days after ingestion: abdominal pains, nausea, vomiting and diarrhoea; with heavily infected meat these symptoms can be especially severe. Later, at the end of the first week, when the larvae begin their migration from the intestinal walls, a profound weakness and lethargy sometimes overcomes the patient. This may be accompanied by a persistent fever, and the larvae, as they invade the voluntary muscles, may bring on sensations of muscular pain, weakness and stiffness.

Fortunately most victims suffer only a minor infection, have only a mild illness and make a slow but steady recovery, eventually losing all symptoms even though the larvae remain encysted in their muscles. More severe cases, however, may be in considerable peril, mortality rates as high as 30 per cent having been recorded in some epidemics. The outlook is in fact considered grave where severe symptoms such as diarrhoea occur within forty-eight hours of eating infected meat. In fatal cases, death usually occurs in the sixth week and is caused by either a form of pneumonia, or chronic weight loss, or else a toxaemic state resembling typhoid.

Trichinosis has been recognized since 1836, but both Andrée and Stefansson may be excused for remaining unaware of its dangers. Not until after the Second World War was it known that Arctic mammals are often heavily infected, a 1947 survey of polar bears in Greenland showing that nearly 30 per cent were carriers. In 1956 a similar survey in Alaska revealed an infection rate of 52·9 per cent, and trichinosis has come to be seen as a major hazard for people living off game meat in Arctic regions.

Dr Tryde's hypothesis was straightforward, the explorers undoubtedly being at risk. At least three or four of the polar bears they killed were most probably infected with trichinella larvae and the explorers ate bear meat practically every day during their march. At times they ate it raw, but even when it was prepared it was probably inadequately cooked. The larvae of *Trichinella spiralis* cannot survive a minimum cooking temperature of 140°C maintained for thirty minutes per pound of meat, but Strindberg, cast in the role of the expedition's cook, had only a primus stove for culinary achievements and a supply of paraffin which needed careful conservation. From trichinosis epidemics reported in temperate climes following the ingestion of undercooked pork, it has been noted that the cook in a household is particularly at risk, given the temptation of sampling 'tasters' of uncooked or partially cooked meat while preparing a meal. Significantly it was Strindberg, the expedition's cook, who was first to die.

In November 1949 Dr Tryde began seriously to investigate his theory, and travelled to Gränna in Sweden, the birthplace of Andrée, where a museum contains the expedition's relics. He made a second visit in January 1950, and this time was allowed to put his theory to the test, taking back to Denmark fourteen tiny fragments of bear meat scraped from the bones of one of the polar bears the explorers had killed. His total sample weighed no more than three grams, yet in Copenhagen he submitted the samples for laboratory examination. On 20 August he received the results: twelve capsules of *Trichinella spiralis* were identifiable in the fourteen minute scraps. Dr Tryde's many findings were duly read to the Eighteenth Session of the Office International des Épizooties in Paris in 1950 as part of a paper presented by his colleague, Dr Hans Roth.

The Tryde theory was elegant as well as attractive, and indeed it fitted practically all the known facts, even though a number of medical authorities have found it difficult to accept. It is, for one thing, far from easy to make any firm diagnosis of trichinosis while relying solely on a description of symptoms. For another, the manifestations of the disease are notably variable and the diaries of the explorers give an incomplete picture. Was it really possible for all three of them to have succumbed to a complaint which normally carries a mortality rate of between 5 and 30 per cent?

The circumstances here, however, were not normal. It does not, in fact, seem implausible to conclude that repeated doses of infected meat would have produced the disease in an exceptionally intensive form, and once that is accepted, it seems easy to visualize the explorers overcome by fever, weakness and agonizing muscle pains, unable to summon the energy or resolve to cope with or record such a totally unforeseen disaster. The subversive parasite, *Trichinella spiralis*, emerges as the prime suspect in any search for the immediate causes of the destruction of Andrée and his colleagues.

But it also seems clear that, however the events which occurred on White Island are interpreted, the primary reasons for the catastrophe have to be sought in Andrée's personality itself. Despite the unquestionable courage of the explorers, it is their naïvety which remains the most astonishing facet of the whole saga. There is an almost heart-breaking innocence which surrounds virtually every aspect of the story.

To begin with, they set out in a balloon which had not been flown in trial flights and, while the endurance record for a balloon journey stood at less than forty-eight hours, confidently expected to remain in flight for perhaps a month. They seemed, moreover, to be totally unaware of the phenomenon of 'false lift' by which a strong wind may suck a balloon upwards from a sheltered launching site, only to deposit it heavily again once it has lifted clear of the windbreak. The lifting power of their balloon was optimistically over-estimated, and if the trailing-lines had not separated immediately at the outset it is doubtful whether the *Örnen* could ever have risen from the waters of the Danes Island harbour. Andrée had spoken publicly of the problem of ice formation on the fabric and rigging, yet he made no allowance for it in his calculations of buoyancy.

Throughout the flight the travellers carefully preserved an immense weight of scientific instruments which had little practical value while cheerfully dumping medicine chests and vital marker buoys overboard as disposable ballast. They even ignored the obvious implications of being forced to jettison their polar buoy, meant to mark the most northerly point of their journey. Once grounded, they hampered their own escape march by obstinately transporting a dumbfound-ing array of impediments, leaving other explorers to marvel at the quantity and nature of the equipment recovered from White Island. They then selected the wrong destination, and finally, at the finish of a march that was practically completed and within sight of home, halted and settled to build a permanent campsite, apparently choosing rather to winter on a bleak, inhospitable Arctic island than to make the last short push for safety and survival.

These ultimately disastrous decisions may all possibly be traced back to Andrée's subconscious need for justification. The pages of his diaries reveal throughout a profound desire for some remarkable achievement, noteworthy exploit or series of observations by which the expedition could be shown to have been worth while. Yet perhaps the most amazing feature remains the fact that they did so nearly succeed despite their miscalculations, mishaps and misjudge-ments, and came within thirty miles of arriving home as heroes. They could not have anticipated the calamity which was to overtake them by such sudden stealth and leave them with only a posthumous glory.

The story of the Andrée expedition is rich in tragic irony – an irony unknowingly underlined by Andrée himself at a point in his diaries where he recorded the following appreciative comment: 'The bear is the Polar-traveller's best friend.'

Chapter 2

The Last Infirmity

In the wake of the Spanish–American War of 1898, the United States undertook the administration of Cuba, guaranteeing the country's independence and placing a large garrison on the island. In terms of political strategy, the US Army had gained a foothold in the Caribbean; in terms of medical fact, it had ventured into a steamy cauldron which brewed one of the world's most dangerous diseases.

On 25 June 1900, the senior 'troubleshooter' of the US Army Medical Corps stepped ashore at Havana harbour. Major Walter Reed, greying, upright and forty-nine years old, was a tightly self-disciplined soldier with a weary face. Yet, despite having made the army his career, he was a doctor who had built up a wide respect as a medical investigator. It seemed to be his fate to find himself posted to the most unsalubrious locations. There had hardly been time for him to complete a massive project to investigate and control the outbreaks of typhoid fever which beset the US military camps in the aftermath of the Spanish–American War before he was dispatched to Cuba.

He arrived, bearing only the vaguest of orders from his superior officer, General George Sternberg, Surgeon-General to the US Army. With his assistant, Acting-Assistant-Surgeon Lieutenant James Carroll, and two other medical officers, he was instructed to set up a commission 'for the purpose of pursuing scientific investigations with reference to the infectious diseases prevalent on the Island of Cuba'. There was, however, little doubt in Reed's mind that he had been sent to Cuba to investigate one disease in particular: yellow fever.

Yellow fever was among the most feared diseases in the western hemisphere, and among the most mystifying. Strangely enough, although it is undoubtedly one of the oldest of the haemorrhagic fevers and has ranked with smallpox and plague as one of the three most lethal killers among the great epidemic diseases, its discovery was relatively recent. Historically speaking, it was something which Columbus and the explorers who followed him stumbled over in the great semi-circle of Caribbean islands making up the Spanish Main. The first European settlement in the New World, which Columbus established in 1492 at Ysabella in Hispaniola, today Isabella in the Dominican Republic, was practically wiped out within ten years of its foundation by tropical disease. At this distance in time, we cannot for certain identify the various epidemics which brought that community low, but yellow fever seems likely to have been among them.

Was the unfamiliar disease *Matlazahuatl*, which Cortés found among the Aztecs of Mexico in 1519, yellow fever; and could the 'Pest of Havana', a lingering scourge which afflicted Cuba in 1620, have been the same infliction? These remain matters for debate by medical historians, but there can be no doubt that the lethal pestilence of 'haemorrhaging black vomit' which, in 1648, swept through the islands of St Kitts, Barbados and Martinique, reaching even as far as the Yucatán peninsula of Mexico, was a yellow-fever epidemic. *El vomito negro* was characteristic of yellow fever at its worst, and its clinical picture was to become only too familiar throughout the West Indies.

The illness seized on its victims with a rapid onset of fever with chills and rigors. The fever then mounted alongside an all-pervading sense of weakness, headache, backache and a slowly increasing soreness in the limbs. Often there was nausea and vomiting, and it was the frequent small gastric haemorrhages occurring in severe cases that led to the appearance of the notorious black vomit. After two or three days passed in a confused, restless nightmare of aching flesh, drenching sweats and limb-shaking chills, there usually followed a deceptive remission. The fever might subside, the aches and pains abate, the flushed, delirious invalid sink into a gentle sleep, awaking to the dawning hope that perhaps the worst was over.

For some it was, and for these fortunate cases a slow but steady convalescence followed, their confidence boosted by knowing that a life-long immunity had been acquired. In other cases, however, the fever, after two or three days of respite, ominously returned, an intense jaundice set in and the dreaded black vomiting reoccurred. Now there was a tendency to episodes of unrestrained bleeding from nose and gums. Blood might appear in the urine, or patches of bleeding occur into the skin. The patient became violent and confused, struggling to rise from the bed and leave the sick-room. Even at this stage it was still possible to recover, but more often than not a feverish coma now led on to convulsions and death.

The most alarming aspect was that a case of yellow fever was rarely an isolated event. One incident presaged an epidemic. Moreover, it was impossible to guess where it kept its lair. It seemed to smoulder undetected in the West Indian heat, the filth and the smells of the island ports, waiting only for the arrival of a fresh cargo of victims to fuel its fires. As a West Indian military report of the seventeenth century commented: 'The arrival of a stranger at almost any time or season in the West Indies was sufficient to develop yellow fever.' The disembarkation of even a hundred soldiers fresh out from Europe was enough to ignite a major outbreak. Sometimes, given good fortune, the illness could masquerade as a mild 'acclimatization fever', but in 1664, on the island of St Lucia, only eighty-nine out of 1,500 soldiers survived.

If the dangers and problems confronting those who disembarked were not enough, the dilemma facing those remaining on ship was worse. With the vessel again at sea, it could be found that the disease had crept aboard. Now yellow fever would strike this way and that among the passengers and crew as it picked its prey from the penned-in victims. Sometimes its selection of cases seemed merely capricious. At other times, it appeared ruthless and insistent, brushing aside precautions and defeating every attempt at isolation. It could also at times give an impression of possessing a sadistic malice as it made its way mockingly from berth to berth along one side of a ship before turning methodically back along the other. Those aboard could then do nothing except watch and wait until, with yellow quarantine flag fluttering, the vessel limped into some unwelcoming harbour.

It happened more often, on the other hand, that the disease would evidently burn itself out during a long voyage, so that by the time a ship reached harbour it would seem free from infection. Nevertheless the fever might now break out anew among the dockers unloading the hold, or those working on the wharfs, and flare within days into a fresh epidemic.

Even those fever-ships that brought no immediate infection to a port could not yet be considered safe. Back at sea, with the vessel launched on a fresh voyage, with even a changed crew and new passengers, the disease might yet re-erupt as murderously as ever. A ship could itself seem haunted by the disease, and so bad did the reputation of certain ships become that individual frigates and transports were abandoned and scuttled in the belief that the miasma of yellow fever clung to their timbers.

In 1668, yellow fever was imported into New York. Striking at a totally unprepared population, the disease leapt from waterfront to dockside taverns, from taverns to houses in the town, until it ran through the whole community. It raged throughout the summer until it seemed that the disease had taken up permanent residence, hiding in alleyways, clinging to walls and rafters as it clung to ships' timbers. Then came winter, its cold rains and biting winds mysteriously wiping the town clean of infection.

In 1691, Boston fell victim; in 1695, Philadelphia; in 1699, Charleston in South Carolina. The entire eastern seaboard of the American continent was at risk. Between 1702 and 1800, thirty-five cities in the United States suffered from outbreaks, and from 1800 the disease visited the country practically every year. Not surprisingly, back in Europe, *el vomito negro* was also a recognized intruder in Spanish ports, even invading French and British harbours. In temperate climates, however, the disease never managed to gain any permanent foothold, whereas in the United States it became one of the most feared diseases, bringing with illness and death an almost total disruption of trade.

Desperate attempts were often made to conceal its presence in a town, physicians and local officials conniving in deception. In 1853, yellow fever attacked New Orleans, causing 29,020 cases with 8,101 deaths, yet the medical profession, the city council and the newspapers all managed to deny the existence of an epidemic until the death rate exceeded 200 a day. In 1878, yellow fever swept up the Mississippi valley, spreading throughout the southern states and reaching as far north as Virginia and St Louis and along the Tennessee River to Chattanooga. There were at least 120,000 cases and 20,000 deaths, and, in his annual message to the nation that year, the President, Rutherford Hayes, remarked how yellow fever had brought 'a loss to the country . . . to be reckoned by the hundreds of millions of dollars'.

From a medical viewpoint, yellow fever was one of the most perplexing diseases. It regarded none of the rules. To start with, although it appeared in catastrophic epidemics, it did not seem to be infectious in the strict sense. Indeed, there was nothing to suggest that it passed from individual to individual. It was quite possible to visit or nurse a sufferer without contracting the disease. In some epidemics, as many as thirty in every 100 of the population were attacked, yet wives who slept beside dying husbands and mothers who hardly left the bedsides of sick children often escaped unscathed.

It was a commonplace observation that the disease clung to a place rather than to a person. Thus there was always the haunting fear that a sufferer could somehow infect his or her surroundings. As certain ships came to be condemned as 'yellow-fever ships', so certain houses came to be regarded as 'yellow-fever houses'. Fresh cases might appear in these dwellings long after the original victim was dead or recovered. It was considered extremely hazardous for a newcomer or non-immune person to visit such a house, especially after dusk. It had been noticed how the disease travelled more easily after daylight faded. Yellow fever was reputed to be a disease of darkness and night, and in Santos and Rio merchants and businessmen might be observed leaving town before sunset as they congregated at the railway station to return to their families safely settled in isolated homes far out in the countryside.

Unsurprisingly, the welter of confused information and folk wisdom produced various interpretations. The 'contagionists' insisted that, like any other infectious disease, yellow fever was conveyed between sufferers. This virtually instinctive attitude led, in time of epidemic, to neighbouring towns imposing fiercely resented quarantine rules upon one another's citizens, and fugitives fleeing infected towns often finding themselves treated with startling inhumanity. At Milford in Delaware State, the inhabitants not only burnt a wagon-load of goods belonging to a lady traveller from fever-struck Philadelphia, but also tarred and feathered their owner.

Logically enough, the 'contagionist' school of thought, which counted the College of Physicians among its adherents, saw the disease as an unfortunate importation from the West Indies, Haiti and Cuba being blamed as the cesspits which repeatedly contaminated the United States. Yet it was also sometimes tartly said that the 'contagionist' theory was supported exclusively by those with no experience of the disease.

The opposing school, the 'non-contagionists', regarded yellow fever as a local phenomenon, a disease produced by spontaneous generation and organic decomposition when the right circumstances of filth, high temperature, moisture and overcrowding came together. In other words, it was a product of environment, a drifting unhealthy miasma which unfortunately infested certain places and buildings. In Memphis, tar barrels were burnt on street corners in an attempt to consume and detoxicate this clinging invisible pollution.

There was much to commend the 'non-contagionists'' point of view. Yellow fever did occur in circumstances of overcrowding and filth, and it did only flourish and propagate itself in hot climates. After all, as had been often observed, a severe frost was sufficient to stop an epidemic in its tracks. It was also widely accepted that the disease had a seasonal incidence, usually breaking into epidemics at times of high humidity after the heavy rains of early autumn. Like a heavy evening mist, yellow fever seemed to prefer low-lying ground and tended to avoid the higher and more exposed parts of a town. It had even been noted that those living in the upper storeys of houses enjoyed a certain protection. When a town was attacked, the epidemic began at a definite focus, several cases occurring simultaneously in one particular quarter, the epidemic afterwards spreading outwards. In several epidemics it had been remarked that the most likely and most rapid direction of advance was downwind, as though the foul miasma was being swept along by prevailing winds. In New York, in 1822, it even proved possible to observe the disease advancing at an average forty feet a day.

Inevitably, a whole spectrum of opinions and theories shaded into one another. The theory most widely accepted which circumvented some of the contradictions was the one which held that the disease was carried by emanations or a contagion arising from patients and clinging to objects. Since this invisible contagion could only be detected by the fact of a person falling ill in its supposed vicinity, the theory implied that any article which had been in contact with a yellow-fever sufferer must be regarded as infectious; and the more intimately it had been in contact, the more dangerous it was considered to be. If the theory was true, then the disease could, of course, be conveyed in baggage or merchandise.

Determined attempts were therefore made to quarantine and disinfect goods and merchandise coming from any port or district where yellow fever was prevalent. When cases of the disease appeared in a town, everything that had been in close contact with victims was burned. As a logical extension to this there followed the wholesale destruction of 'yellow-fever houses', and in Cuba a large part of the town of Siboney was burnt to the ground in an attempt to halt one epidemic. Interestingly enough, the infected objects thought to convey the contagion were referred to as *fomites*, the plural of a Latin word meaning 'tinder'.

The official medical view was neatly summed up by Dr L. S. Tracy in an article in *Popular Science Monthly* in 1878:

Yellow fever occupies a singular position between the contagious and the non-contagious diseases. The poison is not like that of smallpox, directly communicable from a sick person to a well one; but, although the emanations of the sick are connected with the spread of the disease, they seem to require an appropriate nidus in which to germinate and develop. This nidus must be warm and moist, and there the germs, whatever they are, lie and grow, or in some way develop until they are able to migrate.

In due course, a perceptive medical officer of the US Quarantine Service, Dr Henry Carter, contributed one further interesting observation when he remarked on how there was an apparent delay before the surroundings of a yellow-fever patient became infectious to others. Dr Carter had become intrigued by the pattern of cases occurring when yellow fever broke out aboard ships. After an initial case while a ship was in port or within a day or so of its voyage commencing, there would usually be a delay of two to three weeks before other cases began to appear. Allowing for the usual incubation period for yellow fever of four or five days, it must have taken the surroundings ten to fourteen days to grow infectious. In 1897, Henry Carter seized on the opportunity to confirm his ideas when yellow fever attacked Orwood and Taylor, two small towns in northern Mississippi. In the isolated farm-houses and homesteads of these modest communities, he found the very same characteristic pattern of cases as when the disease occurred on shipboard. In one case, a homesteader fell ill on 1 August and was successfully nursed in his own home. Among the eight people who visited him between 6 and 16 August while he was ill, there were no cases of yellow fever; among the thirty-four who visited him after this, thirty-three developed the disease. Carter could only conclude that it took almost two weeks for the homestead to become infectious.

Unfortunately, Henry Carter had one more observation to add from first-hand experience. If ships and houses became infectious, objects such as bales or baggage or pieces of furniture evidently did not. It was practically unknown, he pointed out, for baggage handlers or inspectors in the US Quarantine Service to develop the disease. The cycle of contradiction was complete.

Walter Reed, busy establishing his commission at the Columbia Barracks in Quemados, could not have been unaware that there were pressures at his back. For over two centuries, the West Indies had been seen as the breeding ground for the recurrent invasions of yellow fever which year by year assaulted American cities. Yellow fever was undoubtedly rife in Cuba. In the previous fifty years there had been at least 35,000 deaths from the disease in the city of Havana alone. And now, at last, America had a foothold in the Caribbean and a chance to tackle the pestilence at source. But how was it to do so?

To increase pressures on Walter Reed still further, there was a widespread feeling, not only among the general public but also in the scientific community, that the time was ripe for the problem of yellow fever to be solved. Within the previous few years, new bacteriological techniques had shown the causes of numerous diseases. In this period of great bacteriological discovery a scientist might achieve an international, indeed almost a household reputation, virtually overnight. Yet yellow fever posed as pretty a puzzle as any conundrum under the sun. If it had not been so direly lethal it would have been infuriating.

The army commission began by attempting to isolate and identify the germ that caused yellow fever. At least three different organisms had up till then been cited as the offending bacillus. At the University of Sienna, a plaque had already been unveiled, somewhat prematurely, to commemorate the discovery of the 'yellow-fever germ' by Dr Sanarelli.

For a while, the commission busied itself with a series of autopsies and persistent bacteriological studies, but by the end of July was forced to conclude ruefully that none of the bacteria so far indicted by would-be discoverers could be in any way responsible.

It was a bold pronouncement. Walter Reed and his fellow officers were dismissing in effect not only the claims of Dr Sanarelli of Sienna but also those of their own commanding officer, General Dr George Sternberg, the Surgeon-General of the United States Army who had set up the commission and appointed its members. For thirteen years, General Sternberg had been maintaining on culture plates in his laboratory a bacterium which he had isolated from yellow-fever patients, and Walter Reed must have known in his heart that the underlying purpose of the commission was to substantiate General Sternberg's claim to be the discoverer of the yellow-fever germ.

With detached resolution, however, the commission refuted the general's claim along with every other, but, having thus summarily demolished the notions of all contenders, found itself in the embarrassing position of having nothing to offer in their place. No trace of an offending bacillus could be detected.

Here the commission paused to consider its next step. Either it could continue with an increasingly concentrated search for the germ by examining ever more samples of blood, serum and body fluids from the victims of the disease, or it could launch itself on a bold but unorthodox attempt to solve the strange riddle of yellow fever's mode of spread by direct experiment. With an audacious flourish, the commission chose the second option, but at once found itself face to face with a difficult ethical dilemma. No animal susceptible to yellow fever had yet been discovered, and so all experiments would have to be made on human beings. The nub of the matter lay in the simple fact that, should yellow fever be successfully transmitted to an individual by an experimental procedure, he or she would stand only a 70 per cent chance of survival.

Human experiments had been conducted almost a century earlier, but they were startling and bizarre in design. In 1789, Nathaniel Potter, later to be first Professor of Medicine at the University of Maryland, soaked towels in the 'perspirable matter' of a yellow-fever patient, wrapped them about his own head and retired to bed. Despite the 'extreme nauseous foetor', he slept until seven in the morning and suffered no ill-effects. Subsequently he tried to inoculate himself with the same material. Thirteen years after that, a young medical student, Stubbins Ffirth, from the University of Philadelphia, took matters a good deal further. During the Philadelphia epidemics of 1802 and 1803, he deposited black vomit and blood into cuts made in his arms and legs. He administered black vomit to animals and inhaled the fumes from six ounces of 'bloody material' which he heated over a sandbath in a small room. The residue of 'bloody material' he made into pills and swallowed. He then tried inoculating himself with infected blood, serum, saliva, perspiration, bile and urine. The fact that Mr Ffirth survived his experiments unharmed can only be explained in retrospect by assuming either that he was already immune or that he was mistaken in the diagnosis of the patient from whom he took his samples.

The members of the yellow-fever commission, undaunted by the risks and complex ethical problems, resolved to act as their own first guinea-pigs. It was perhaps unfortunate that as soon as the decision was taken, their chairman, the leading hero in the drama, should have been recalled to Washington to put the finishing touches to his report on typhoid fever. Walter Reed's most trusted assistant, James Carroll, was therefore left in charge of the experiments and field-work.

Carroll was an experienced, accomplished bacteriologist who had worked with Reed over several years. A colleague once described him as 'a bald-headed, bespectacled man with a light-red moustache, projecting ears and a rather dull expression', remarking that he was a 'not very entertaining person' and that he had 'a narrow horizon'. Despite his plainness and lack of social grace, however, he was an unusual individual. Born south of the Thames at Woolwich, he emigrated to Canada at the age of fifteen. Here he lived as a backwoodsman, working in a variety of jobs, such as lumberjack, blacksmith's assistant and railroad labourer. At the age of twenty he drifted into the US Army, and thirteen years later managed to combine the role of part-time student with army duties. He qualified as a doctor at thirty-seven, finding himself uncomfortable and self-conscious in his new social station. He was now forty-six years old.

As a first step the commission sought a meeting with an elderly local physician, Dr Carlos Finlay of Havana. For the past twenty years, Dr Finlay had been claiming to have solved the mystery of yellow fever's mode of spread. He was quite convinced that the disease was carried from victim to victim by mosquitoes acting like so many tiny flying syringes. Yet while Dr Finlay had made over a hundred determined attempts to transmit yellow fever from one person to another by the agency of carefully reared mosquitoes, he had produced no case of the disease and so absolutely no evidence to support his remarkable claims. In local medical circles, his theories were politely dismissed as the harmless foibles of an elderly physician.

It was only twenty years since Sir Patrick Manson had demonstrated that the tropical disease filariasis (elephantiasis) was transmitted by mosquitoes, and so had become the first scientist to show that disease could be insect borne. It was less than three years since Ronald Ross had proved that malaria was conveyed by the same insects, though it had taken Ross, working in India, over two and a half years and the dissection of thousands of gnats and mosquitoes to unmask the carrier of the malarial parasite. And now here was Dr Carlos Finlay with his mind already made up, on the basis of no confirmatory evidence, that yellow fever was conveyed by one particular species of mosquito: a common house-mosquito then known as *Culex fasciatus*.

The members of the commission were nevertheless inclined to take an alert interest in Dr Finlay's ideas. The old doctor showed Carroll and another member of the commission, Jesse Lazear, a small bowl of water in which some tiny cigar-shaped eggs clung to the side, half in, half out of the water. These were the eggs of the mosquito, and he had found that they could dry and blow about in the wind for several weeks until, as soon as they were moistened by the warm rain, their process of development began. Only the female mosquito needed to suck blood, and then only when about to lay her eggs. Without such a meal of blood, her eggs would be infertile. Dr Finlay could visualize the female mosquito taking blood from a yellow-fever victim, but there his vision faltered. Did the long needle-like proboscis of the female mosquito then carry the germs to the next victim, rather as a 'dirty' unsterilized hypodermic needle might carry sepsis, or did the mosquito, sickened after its contaminated meal, fall into water which, in turn, poisoned anyone who drank it? With remarkable generosity, Dr Finlay donated his entire stock of *Culex fasciatus* eggs to the commission.

The task of hatching mosquitoes from Dr Finlay's supply of eggs was entrusted to the third member of the commission, Jesse Lazear. In many ways, Lazear was in sharp contrast to his senior colleague, Carroll. He was thirty-three years old, a handsome young doctor who seemed one of fortune's favoured sons. Born in Baltimore, he graduated from Columbia before taking up an internship at Bellevue Hospital in New York. From there he went to Europe and the Pasteur Institute for further training. On his return, he held a teaching appointment at the Johns Hopkins Hospital as assistant resident physician, sharing in some notable research work by Osler and Thayer on the malarial parasite. Thayer found him 'quiet, retiring, modest almost to a fault . . . yet a manly man with a good vigorous temper, well controlled'.

Lazear's experience of malarial research had turned him into an excellent entomologist, and it was this which made him most valuable to the commission. His evolved method of using mosquitoes was quite simple. They were hatched in captivity and allowed to bite human beings only under controlled conditions. A mosquito selected for an experiment would be trapped in a large test-tube which was then placed mouth down against the forearm or abdomen of the human subject, allowing the mosquito to settle on the skin and insert its proboscis. Once its meal was over, a gentle tap on the glass made the insect fly up into the top of the test-tube which could then be removed complete with occupant.

The experiment now would consist in letting a mosquito feed, first, on a yellow-fever patient, then on a non-immune volunteer; and there was no shortage of yellow-fever patients. In Cuba, the yellow-fever season ran from late June until the end of November. It was now mid August, and, as if to mock the unrelenting efforts of the sanitary squads of the American Quarantine Service, the disease was taking a terrible toll among the non-immune soldiers of the American garrison. The Military Governor of Havana had died quite early in the epidemic, followed shortly by the commissary officer. When the latter died, his wife, having travelled from Cincinnati to reach him, shot herself and was buried with him. Within days, the quartermaster-sergeant was dead, as well as the American superintendent of the San José Asylum. At Quemados, the Las Animas Hospital, where the yellow-fever cases were nursed, was full.

On 11 August, the commission made its first attempts to transmit the disease. Lazear allowed mosquitoes that had bitten yellow-fever patients to feed on the skin of his own arm. The mosquitoes were also applied to the arms of another medical officer and seven further volunteers. A tense wait set in. Should all nine of the volunteers develop the disease, there was a risk that at least two or three of them would die.

By now the members of the commission were well disposed to the idea that yellow fever could be conveyed by mosquitoes. It offered a neat explanation for both its seasonal and geographical incidence. Within a few days, however, it became clear that the experiment had failed: none of the subjects showed the slightest sign of sickening.

A conflicting mixture of consternation and relief followed. Even though his own attempts to perform the experiment had failed over a hundred times, Dr Carlos Finlay was shaken and subdued, searching vainly for some fault in the experimental design. In the laboratory, Carroll and Lazear laboured on, but an air of disappointment and uncertainty hung over their work. Lazear now felt considerable doubts about the role of mosquitoes, but nevertheless continued to look after the insects meticulously. Each one was kept isolated in the laboratory, carefully sealed by a small plug of cottonwool inside its own wide-bore test-tube. He spent long mornings at Las Animas Hospital, trying to induce his charges to settle on and to take blood from yellow-fever victims. He even spent the whole of the morning of 27 August trying to persuade one particular mosquito to feed. It seemed weak and tired, and he feared that, without nourishment, it would die. After lunch, both Carroll and Lazear tried again, placing the insect in turns upon their own arms until, at last, it settled and took blood from Carroll.

In the late afternoon of 31 August, Carroll developed an unpleasant throbbing headache while swimming with his fellow officers. By 8 p.m. he was in the yellow-fever ward. It was four days since he had fed the mosquito.

There was immediate consternation. Lazear's records showed that the mosquito which bit Carroll had fed on a succession of yellow-fever patients, ranging from a severe case, bitten twelve days previously, to a mild case, bitten only two days earlier. Both Lazear and the fourth member of the commission, Aristide Agramonte, were now convinced that the mosquito had transmitted yellow fever to their colleague, but unfortunately his sudden illness proved nothing. There had been cases of the disease scattered throughout Havana with whom Carroll had been in contact. During the incubation period for his illness, Carroll had gone not only into Havana but into the yellow-fever wards at Las Animas, even into the autopsy room. He could have caught the disease anywhere.

In a desperate attempt to retrieve a semblance of scientific validity, Lazear decided that the accidental experiment must be repeated: the mosquito which had bitten Carroll must be persuaded to bite again, but this time to infect a subject who had had no chance of contracting the disease elsewhere. A trooper from the Seventh Cavalry was the volunteer. He had never been in the tropics before, and had not left the military reservation for nearly two months. There had been no possible contact with yellow fever. Within three days of his mosquito bite, the trooper fell ill. Lazear felt both horrified and relieved.

From now on, the members of the commission were to experience the full anguish of human experiments, from the viewpoint of both subject and investigator. Carroll grew desperately sick. A visiting physician, shocked by his appearance, described him 'lying in a state of prostration, his face flushed with a high fever, his eyes bloodshot, his restless body tossing on the bed'. As he lapsed in and out of a fevered confusion, Carroll struggled desperately to impress on those about him that the disease had been given him by a mosquito. His nurse dutifully recorded in his case records: 'Says he got his illness from the bite of a mosquito – delirious!'

Lazear and Agramonte were by now beside themselves with anxiety. Lazear tried to assuage his sense of guilt by consoling himself that Carroll had placed the mosquito on his arm himself. Walter Reed, the absentee chairman, struggled to complete his typhoid report in Washington while trying to keep track of events in Cuba by letter and cable. He had seen at once that Carroll's illness proved nothing. Now he wrote, pleading for news. Their one relief from worry came from the fact that the trooper from the Seventh Cavalry was suffering only a mild attack.

Carroll's condition grew critical. On the third day, at the height of his fever, having been given a mustard foot-bath and covered in heavy grey army blankets, he suffered what later medical authorities regard as an episode of acute dilation of the heart. In his own words, he 'felt a sudden pain and embarrassment at the heart. The pain was very acute and accompanied with a feeling of distension, as if the organ was much distended and being arrested in diastole. Happily, it lasted but a few moments.' Yet by 7 September his condition was improving, and on the 13th he was allowed to leave his bed for the first time.

From Washington, Walter Reed wrote a letter of jubilant relief. His work on the typhoid report was now complete and he began to make plans to return to Cuba. In Havana, the morale of the commission recovered. Carroll, Lazear and Agramonte were all convinced that they now had a grip on a tangible lead.

Then, on 18 September, five days after Carroll was allowed to get up, Jesse Lazear was seized with a chill. A few hours later he had another and was obviously developing a fever. Carroll, still weak, twice examined samples of Lazear's blood for malarial parasites, and when the results were negative reluctantly advised that his colleague be admitted to the yellow-fever ward. Before he would agree, however, Lazear insisted on handing over his laboratory records to Carroll.

For the first few days, Lazear seemed to hold his own, but then began to suffer bouts of retching, bringing up the dreaded black vomit of a full-blown case of classical yellow fever. He was fully aware of the import of the symptom. 'I shall never forget', Carroll wrote later, 'the expression of alarm in his eyes when I last saw him alive in the third or fourth day of his illness. The spasmodic contractions of his diaphragm indicated that black vomit was impending, and he fully appreciated their significance.'

His nurse wrote how

the black vomit would spurt from his mouth up through the bars of his cot. I had just relieved the day nurse and gone on for the night; my efforts to keep him in bed failed and I called for help, but before assistance reached me he had made several turns round the room in his efforts to get out. All night it took two men to hold him . . .

Lazear died on 28 September, leaving, without financial support, a wife, a small son and a baby daughter he had never seen.

But the commission's grief at the loss of their colleague was overshadowed by the urgent need to establish how he became infected. A desperate search through his laboratory notes showed no record of Lazear ever having exposed himself to further experimental mosquito bites, yet, as he handed over the records to Carroll, he had confided in his colleague that he attributed his illness to a chance happening while working on the wards at Las Animas. On 13 September, when he was applying mosquitoes to yellow-fever patients, five days before he fell ill, an insect flying about the ward settled on the back of his hand. He recognized it at once as one of the common house-mosquitoes, present in the hospital in large numbers. Not wanting to disturb the insect in the test-tube which he was holding against a patient's abdomen, he had not brushed it away but had allowed it to bite and take its fill.

Walter Reed got back to Cuba on 3 October, Carroll having been given orders to disinfect Lazear's laboratory to make it safe for the chairman to work there. He found his commission sadly depleted: Lazear dead, Agramonte on leave in the

United States, Carroll anxious for sick-leave. Carroll was clearly disgruntled. In the privacy of letters to his wife he accused Reed of cowardice. A fellow officer had jokingly suggested that Reed should be accused of running away. 'I thought to myself you have no idea how nearly you have come to the truth,' wrote Carroll. 'My friend will be as brave as a lion now that the yellow-fever season is about over and he will take particular care not to take the same chances I did.'

Reed, himself, seems to have felt reservations about his role in events. 'I have been so ashamed of myself for being in a safe country, while my associates have been coming down with yellow fever,' he wrote. In a later letter he remarked: 'Perhaps I owe my life to my departure from Cuba, for being an old man, I might have been quickly carried off.' His commanding officer, General Sternberg, suggested he should not return to Cuba, but Reed had replied that 'as the senior member of a Board investigating yellow fever, my place is in Cuba as long as the work goes on'. He did agree, however, to take every precaution and not 'with the facts we now have to allow a *loaded* mosquito to bite'.

Reed stayed in Cuba just ten days, studying Lazear's laboratory records and preparing a draft report. He was convinced he had solved the riddle of yellow fever's mode of spread. Of eleven volunteers bitten by mosquitoes, two had developed yellow fever. For Reed, it was enough: yellow fever was conveyed by mosquitoes.

On 13 October, Walter Reed left Cuba, bound for Indianapolis and the annual meeting of the American Public Health Association. On 23 October, he rose to address the 150 delegates and spoke for forty minutes. Almost simultaneously, a short report, written by Reed, citing Carroll, Agramonte and the departed Lazear as co-authors, was published in the *Philadelphia Medical Journal*. Meanwhile, back in Washington, DC, General Sternberg was already associating his own name with the discovery.

The first triumphant claim had thus been made, but the matter was hardly settled. The preliminary communication to the American Public Health Association was based on only two cases: those of Carroll and the trooper from the Seventh Cavalry. One of these had been accidental and proved very little; the other had led only to a mild bout of yellow fever, the very mildness of the trooper's symptoms leaving the diagnosis open to dispute. Unfortunately, Lazear's fatal attack was inadmissible evidence. There was nothing to prove how he acquired his infection. Further studies were needed.

On 8 November, Reed returned to Cuba with resources at his disposal to establish a temporary army medical centre where the yellow-fever commission could complete its work in ideal conditions. Within twenty-four hours he had chosen as its campsite, about a mile from Quemados, an isolated uncultivated field in the countryside. Work began at once on erecting the seven large hospital tents and two timber-frame buildings which were to make up its accommodation. By 20 November, all was ready, the centre having been christened Camp Lazear.

The camp was essentially an isolation hospital, designed to protect its inmates, the subjects of experimental procedures, from any accidental contact with yellow fever. It was a rule of the camp that every non-immune individual should have pulse and temperature recorded three times a day so that any intrusion of the disease might be detected at once.

The project was working against the clock. The yellow-fever season was practically over, and most of the mosquitoes reared from Dr Carlos Finlay's stock of eggs were dead. It was at this moment that the weather chose to break. A storm struck Cuba, uprooting trees and destroying the mosquitoes by blowing them many miles out to sea. In haste, Reed led a small party of medical officers on a mosquito egg hunt, rummaging among the tin-cans and broken pottery thrown out on the rubbish dumps, examining any object which might contain stagnant water. The party's determination was rewarded when they found an abundant supply of eggs floating in foul cans which had, for want of sewers, been used as toilets.

The programme of research at Camp Lazear fell into two parts. The first was designed to confirm and extend the commission's original mosquito studies; the second to determine whether yellow fever could be conveyed by *fomites* – objects such as clothing and bedding which had been in contact with patients.

With some trepidation, the commission resumed work by repeating earlier experiments. On 5 December, a volunteer private from Ohio was subjected to bites from infected mosquitoes. On 8 December, he fell ill. Walter Reed watched, with fascination, the first case of experimentally induced yellow fever he had ever seen.

During the next week, the experiment was repeated four times, producing three further cases. In contrast with Dr Finlay's repeated failures, the experiment was now achieving a success rate of 80 per cent. Reed, excited and triumphant, wrote in a report:

It can readily be imagined that the occurrence of four cases of yellow fever in our small command of twelve non-immunes, within the space of one week, while giving rise to feelings of exultation in the hearts of the experimenters, in view of the vast importance attaching to the results, might inspire quite other sentiments in the bosoms of those who had previously consented to submit themselves to the mosquito's bite. In fact, several of our good-natured Spanish friends, who had jokingly compared our mosquitoes to 'the little flies that buzzed harmlessly about their tables', suddenly appeared to lose all interest in the progress of science, and forgetting for the moment even their own personal aggrandisement, incontinently severed their connection with Camp Lazear. Personally, while lamenting to some extent their departure, I could not but feel that in placing themselves beyond our control they were exercising the soundest judgement.

It was a decision he had already taken himself.

With the commission's continuing experiments, the final pieces of the jigsaw fell into place. A case of yellow fever was evidently infectious only during the first few days of illness. Any mosquito which bit the sufferer during this phase would become infected. But even as there was an incubation period in man, so, it turned out, there was an incubation period in mosquitoes. The crucial factor was that a delay of almost two weeks intervened between the moment when the mosquito took its contaminated meal and its becoming infectious.

Henry Carter, the medical officer for the US Quarantine Service, had estimated on between ten and seventeen days before the surroundings of a yellow-fever victim became infectious. The commission's studies indicated that it took between nine and sixteen days before an infected mosquito was capable of transmitting the disease. The match was remarkable.

Thus had the external incubation period of the disease in the mosquito defeated Dr Carlos Finlay, and thus were the failure of his repeated attempts to prove his theory and the commission's lack of success with its own first trial both explained. So far as the commission could now make out, once a mosquito became infectious it remained a yellow-fever carrier for life.

Hence it was not miasma but mosquitoes which haunted

the yellow-fever houses, the doom-laden ships. It was the late-evening swarms of mosquitoes that percolated through the low-lying areas of the town and failed to rise to the first-floor apartments. This was why yellow fever only flourished in hot climates and why the worst epidemic could be stopped in its tracks by the onset of a sharp cold spell. The hot rainy season conversely ushered in the yellow-fever season, since it was the warm rain that hatched out the mosquitoes. Burning tar barrels and quarantining travellers' baggage could hardly be expected to stop the spread of the disease. Such precautions were as useless as trying to halt the wind.

There remained the question of whether *fomites* could convey the disease, and determined efforts were made to convert one of the timber-framed buildings into a 'yellow-fever house'. The building was basically one large room, ventilated only by two small windows, both facing south. The windows were closed by the usual wire screens, and also by glass sashes on the inside and wooden shutters on the outside, the latter being kept tightly closed to exclude day-light. Throughout the experiments, the room was heated to maintain a constant temperature of about 94°F and a high humidity. Entrance to the hut was through a double door with a screened vestibule, for the only intruders the commission sought to exclude from the environment were mosquitoes.

As soon as this dark, overheated room was ready for occupation, three large boxes, filled with sheets, pillowcases and blankets, were brought from Las Animas Hospital. The linen, taken from the beds of yellow-fever victims, was soiled with black vomit, urine and faecal discharges. It had been deliberately further contaminated, packed into the boxes and stored for two weeks, a period long enough to allow the 'yellow-fever poison' to ferment and proliferate. Three non-immune volunteers now unpacked the boxes. They shook the contents about in the hot close atmosphere, used some of the linen to make up their beds and hung the rest about the room in an attempt to contaminate the air.

For three weeks, the volunteers slept each night in those same beds, using the stained 'comfortable' sheets and blankets, although sometimes the stench was so strong it drove them retching from the hut. During daylight hours, they were allowed to leave the room and live in the isolation of an adjacent tent, dining by way of consolation off the choicest meals the army could provide. The whole experiment was repeated four times with a succession of volunteers, some of whom even slept in unwashed nightshirts previously worn by yellow-fever patients. And none of these volunteers developed the slightest trace of disease.

To prove its point beyond argument, the commission now set out to convert the second timber-framed hut into a 'yellow-fever house', this time using its own mosquito theory as a basis. In the second building, the single well-lit room was divided into two compartments by a wire-screen partition that allowed air to circulate freely between each half but excluded the passage of insects such as mosquitoes. Beds, made up with freshly laundered sheets and bedding sterilized by steam, were placed in both compartments. Mosquitoes fed on yellow-fever patients were now released into one compartment, and a non-immune soldier who volunteered to enter was bitten almost at once. Within four days, he developed the disease, though he had spent in the hut only three brief periods, each about twenty minutes long. Three non-immune subjects who lived in the other compartment, breathing the same air and sharing identical surroundings but protected from mosquitoes, remained obstinately healthy.

As a final step, the commission attempted to emulate the

mosquito's role by taking blood from yellow-fever patients by hypodermic needle and injecting it directly under the skin of a volunteer. The experiment, repeated four times, produced on each occasion a yellow-fever case within four to five days.

The 1901 annual meeting of the Pan-American Congress was held in Havana, and on 6 February Walter Reed presented to the convention a report on the commission's work. His address was well received, but if he had expected unqualified acclaim he was disappointed. Many physicians felt that mosquitoes could not possibly account for all the cases of yellow fever that occurred. Others, arguing in similar vein, were unable to discount the possibility that *fomites* might still play an important part in transmission. They considered it would be unwise to abandon the quarantining of goods and baggage. There even followed a heated dispute about the identification of the species of mosquito the commission had used. A more serious attack on Reed, however, was based on his having used human beings for experiments, even though the twenty-three volunteers who developed yellow fever at Camp Lazear had all survived. But the most forthright opposition came from a large body of delegates who repeatedly pointed out the commission's lack of success in identifying a specific micro-organism as the germ of yellow fever. In these critics' eyes the commission had failed, and Reed had no answer for them.

Several months later it was brought to Reed's attention that two German researchers, Löffler and Frosch, had just shown how foot-and-mouth disease in cattle was caused by a germ so small it could be passed through the pores of a porcelain filter – in other words, by a germ too small to be seen by a microscope. In August 1901, James Carroll returned to Cuba to repeat the commission's injection experiments. His work was now hampered by official doubts about its safety, but he managed to show how blood from yellow-fever patients remained infectious even after being passed through the finest porcelain filter. On his own initiative, he demonstrated how the infected blood lost all danger as an injection if first heated to 55°C for ten minutes. The conclusion was inescapable: the germ of yellow fever, like that of bovine foot-and-mouth, belonged to a previously unrecognized group of organisms, the ultra-microscopic viruses.

The final vindication of the commission's theories came with their application when the chief sanitary officer of Havana, Surgeon-Major William Gorgas, compelled by duty rather than any whole-hearted support for the commission's views, set about breaking the chain of infection by preventing mosquitoes from reaching yellow-fever sufferers. The sanitary regulations now demanded not only that every case of yellow fever be reported and quarantined, but that sick-rooms be protected by wire screens to exclude mosquitoes. Burning sulphur or pyrethrum was moreover to be used to fumigate every room in an infected house and even in adjacent buildings, so the stupefied insects could be swept up and buried. Sanitary squads concentrated on interrupting the breeding cycle of the mosquito by draining, wherever possible, every collection of stagnant water, or else coating surfaces with a protective film of oil to prevent mosquito eggs being laid or hatched.

Within ninety days of the anti-mosquito campaign commencing, Havana was free of yellow fever for the first time in 150 years. In 1900, a mild year for the disease by Cuban standards, there had been 1,236 cases with 311 deaths; 1901, the year the measures were introduced, saw thirty-one cases with six deaths; in 1902, the disease did not occur in the city.

The results were impossible to ignore. Within two years William Gorgas was sent to Panama, where the attempt made by the French in the 1880s to unite the Atlantic and Pacific oceans by constructing a canal through the isthmus had failed largely because of the difficulty of maintaining a healthy labour force. Each year at least 200 in every 1,000 of their construction workers died from such tropical diseases as malaria or yellow fever. Now it was the United States which took up the challenge, and it was the anti-mosquito campaigns, set in motion by Gorgas, which reduced the death rate to seventeen in every 1,000 and allowed the Panama Canal to be ready for its official opening in 1913. It now seemed possible to contemplate eliminating yellow fever from the whole North American continent and the Caribbean.

As so often happens with intricate, long-standing puzzles, once the first clue had been seized upon, unravelled and understood, the rest, in due course, fell into place. In 1927 it was discovered that yellow fever could be transmitted to rhesus monkeys and certain other animals, so long as these creatures came from a continent where yellow fever was not present. Now yellow fever could be experimented with freely, and, although two eminent bacteriologists died from accidental infections, before long the germ of the disease had been isolated and studied. It proved to be one of the smallest of viruses, only 20 millimicrons or 0·00002 of a millimetre in diameter.

At this point, it was recognized somewhat belatedly that yellow fever was also endemic in tropical Africa, which raised the question of from which side of the Atlantic the disease originated. Certain medical historians now inclined to the view that the West Indies purchased yellow fever along with its slaves. Virtually side by side with these controversies there came the realization that yellow fever was rife among wild monkeys in both the American and African continents. Bacteriologists were disconcerted to find that infection could be transmitted from animals to human beings and that this could be done by more than one variety of mosquito. There was therefore a sylvan cycle as well as an urban cycle to yellow fever, and, given such a huge reservoir of infection in the animal kingdom, no chance of the disease ever being completely eradicated.

In 1937, a vaccine was developed which proved to be one of the most effective vaccines in the world. Between 1940 and 1947, the Rockefeller Foundation produced over 28 million doses at a cost of 2.2 cents a dose, distributing it free to thirty-five tropical countries and agencies. Today the dangers of yellow fever are largely contained, though the persistence of the virus in the wildlife of the jungle canopies poses a continuing threat to man. Sporadic tropical epidemics still occur.

In 1966, with the co-operation of the Cuban government, Camp Lazear was preserved as a memorial to the yellow-fever commission and its work, and to the volunteers who risked their lives. Yet, for the members of the commission who started it all, their triumph proved bitter-sweet. For Aristide Agramonte, the son of an insurgent Cuban general killed in battle, there was an appointment to the chair of bacteriology and experimental pathology in the Medical Faculty at Havana, and a retreat into academic obscurity. For James Carroll, the assistant who bore the brunt of the commission's day-to-day administration, undertook the main burden of the experimental work, even experienced the first attack of artificially induced yellow fever, there was mainly disillusion and the realization that a valve in his heart was irretrievably damaged by the episode of acute cardiac dilation which occurred during his bout of illness. Although his continuing studies and wide knowledge of the subject were to make him a respected authority on the disease, he was never promoted beyond first lieutenant. He did, however, in 1902, succeed Walter Reed as professor of bacteriology and pathology at the Army Medical School in Washington, combining this with the chair of bacteriology and pathology at Columbia University. In 1907, barely six years after his return from Cuba, Carroll died from heart disease at the age of fifty-three.

For Walter Reed, chairman of the committee, there was aggravation and dispute. He was constantly aware of the way his chief, General George Sternberg, was claiming a major role in the discovery, the surgeon-general having managed to convince himself that he set up the commission especially to investigate the role of the mosquito in transmitting yellow fever. Reed even came to resent a newspaper interview from Havana, in which William Gorgas gave a measure of praise to Dr Carlos Finlay. Gorgas wrote, in answer to an angry letter from Reed:

I do not 'honey fuggle the simpering old idiot' a bit. I think he is an old trump as modest as he is kindly and true. His reasoning for selecting the Stegmyia [the house mosquito] as the bearer of yellow fever is the best piece of logical reasoning that can be found in medicine anywhere. I acknowledge that the less . . . said about his experiments . . . the better for the old Doctor's reputation as a scientist.

But if he was conciliatory to Reed in private, in public Gorgas made his own bid for a slice of glory. In his account of the campaign against yellow fever in Cuba he wrote:

Neither the Reed Board, nor any of its members had anything to do with the practical working out of the methods whereby their theory was demonstrated and by means of which yellow fever was finally eliminated from Havana.

Walter Reed did not live to see either the end of the

backbiting or to receive the promotion to colonel for which his name was proposed. On 23 November 1902, just twenty-one months after the commission finished its work, he died, following an operation for appendicitis. He was fifty-one years old.

In 1909, a large general hospital for the army was named after him, and in 1923 the Walter Reed Army Medical Center was opened. It included the Walter Reed Army Institute of Research, the Corps' historical department and several specialized units. It was therefore to Walter Reed that posterity awarded the accolades, but it is clear that every one of those involved in the yellow-fever saga had been driven by a desire for recognition and international renown. The spur had been fame, 'the last infirmity of noble minds'.

Chapter 3

The Case of the Epping Jaundice

The town of Epping in Essex is of Saxon origin, its name meaning 'upland dwellers'. It lies no more than seventeen miles to the north-east of London, but has remained self-contained, the 6,000 acres or so that survive of the former vast and ancient forest of Epping acting as a buffer between it and London's inner suburbs. Even so, its atmosphere is that of a suburban commuter town, with its single long high street of modern shop fronts, its church built between 1889 and 1909 and its population of about 12,000 souls. 'There are few houses of individual merit,' says the architectural historian Nikolaus Pevsner in his Essex volume of the *Buildings of England* series. Nevertheless it is tidy and pleasant if unremarkable. Certainly it gives no sign of having the right to possess its own unique disease, and that it does so is a result of events which occurred in the year 1965.

The first indication of anything amiss came on Monday morning, 8 February, when a consultant physician, Dr Harry Kopelman, began his ward round at Epping's St Margaret's Hospital. One of the six medical students expected to accompany him was missing. On Tuesday the missing medical student turned up, and after asking Dr Kopelman for a consultation told a story which carried some puzzling aspects.

The young man, a 23-year-old student at the London

Hospital Medical College, lived with his wife in Harrow, nearly thirty miles away, having joined Dr Kopelman's unit as recently as 1 February to pick up experience. On Friday evening he felt normal when he returned to Harrow for the weekend, but by Saturday evening had fallen ill with severe pains spreading across the top of his abdomen. The pains seemed to begin below the ribs on the right-hand side and to spread not only across his stomach but up into his chest. They were intermittent, and his family doctor, finding little to account for them, suspected a simple case of indigestion. Yet by 9.30 the pains were so intense that an ambulance was called and the student taken to the casualty department of a local hospital. Again he was examined and again nothing could be found. He was sent home with a diagnosis of 'acute gastritis', and the wife, anxious and puzzled, suffered a mild discomfort across her upper abdomen in apparent sympathy with her husband.

The young man's pains, however, continued throughout the night and the whole of Sunday. By Monday they were at last subsiding, though the student felt ill and extremely tired. Thus on Tuesday, with something of an effort, he travelled the thirty miles to Epping and found Dr Kopelman willing to take the matter rather more seriously than the doctors before him.

The student was certainly quite ill. He was feverish, with a temperature of 37·4°C (99°F), his abdomen was tender to the touch beneath the ribs on the right-hand side, but, most striking of all, his skin was turning yellow; in other words, jaundice was setting in. Dr Kopelman arranged for his admission to hospital, already aware of something odd which did not quite fit with the patterns a doctor expects to find in any onset of jaundice.

Jaundice is not a disease but a symptom which may arise

from one among many causes. In the normal course of events, the liver produces the substance called bile, and during the process extracts the bile pigments from the bloodstream. The function of bile is to assist in breaking down and absorbing fats, and to do its work it has to be passed down the bile duct to the gall-bladder and the part of the intestine called the duodenum. Jaundice occurs when this process is interrupted and the yellow bile pigments build up in the bloodstream and body tissues, possible reasons ranging from liver damage caused by infection to poison or a growth, or to obstruction of the bile duct by a gallstone.

There is an inherently dramatic quality in jaundice as a symptom, even the most experienced doctor finding something deeply curious about the sight of a patient slowly turning yellow. The story which the student told Harry Kopelman was, however, unusual for one reason in particular. It suggested, if anything, a violent colic or pain caused by a gallstone passing down from the gall-bladder to block the main bile duct. But gallstones are an affliction of the middle-aged, and in a young man of twenty-three would be quite noteworthy.

Dr Kopelman resigned himself to await the test results, and that afternoon, while the student's first blood samples were being examined in the laboratories, travelled to the nearby town of Harlow to conduct a weekly out-patient clinic at the Princess Alexandra Hospital. He had scarcely arrived before his medical assistant there, a local general practitioner, sought his advice. His wife, also a doctor – an anaesthetist, in fact – had just fallen ill and was showing signs of jaundice. During the evening Dr Kopelman called at the couple's home and for the second time that day found himself confronting what seemed to be an episode of acute gallstone colic in a young adult.

The coincidence was too remarkable to be ignored. With a certain foreboding, Dr Kopelman contacted another local general practitioner to ask if he was noticing any unusual cases of jaundice in Epping. 'As a matter of fact', his colleague replied, 'there is a funny sort of jaundice going around. I've six cases at the moment!'

Armed with their doctor's consent, Dr Kopelman set out to visit all six cases, but at each step he took the circumstances grew steadily more bizarre. To begin with, he found himself visiting not six houses but three, the cases occurring in pairs, husband and wife sharing the illness in three entirely different households of this one small town. The second startling aspect was the type of house being visited: not poorer, overcrowded homes where infection might be expected to spread rapidly, but the pleasant, spacious residences of professional men and women – the houses of bank managers and executives. It seemed a kind of jaundice that went with wall-to-wall carpeting, accomplished flower arrangements and two cars in the garage.

By now Dr Kopelman had reached the conclusion that nothing made sense. Epping was evidently being visited by a strange illness which fitted no recognized pigeon-holes. The moment had arrived to alert the community physician.

Dr Isidore Ash, Medical Officer of Health for the area, was also growing aware of something rather odd in the making. In one particular respect Harlow Health District, which administered the community health services for Epping and the surrounding villages, was ahead of its time. Infectious hepatitis, a common viral infection which causes jaundice by attacking the liver, was already classified there as a notifiable disease. Dr Ash therefore knew that so far as jaundice went there suddenly seemed to be a good deal of it about. Several cases in Harlow, the main town of the area, all seemed like cases of straightforward virus infection. He was puzzled, however, by a message from a doctor in the village of Chipping Ongar, seven miles east of Epping, some rather unusual cases of jaundice having just turned up there. No sooner had Dr Ash promised to visit them than Harry Kopelman came through on the phone.

Following a hasty conversation, during which they exchanged their various scraps of information, Dr Kopelman returned to his patients and Dr Ash set out for Chipping Ongar, his senses of curiosity and urgency equally heightened. Within the hour he knew that he had come upon further cases of the puzzling disease eventually to be known as the 'Epping jaundice'.

As the community physician, Dr Ash's task was to consider this outbreak overall. He was more concerned with the prevention and control of an epidemic than with individual cases. His department administered a wide area, but all the sufferers so far recognized were linked to this relatively small district: the small town of Epping, the nearby village of Chipping Ongar and the tiny villages and hamlets in the surrounding countryside. A strangely selective illness seemed to have erupted in a particular corner of Essex with virtually explosive suddenness, and the community physician carried an ultimate responsibility for efforts to contain it. His first priority was to define the cause.

There is an old medical adage: listen to the patient, he is telling you what is wrong with him! Dr Ash now needed to listen intently to each patient to sift out the common factor in their stories and so identify the as yet unrecognized and apparently insignificant detail linking them. By comparison and cross-reference, he now needed to seek the elusive but active danger which had reached out to disrupt the lives of each widely separated couple. Looking for a needle in a haystack was an appropriate simile.

At St Margaret's Hospital Dr Kopelman meanwhile found himself admitting the wife of the young medical student, who, after arriving from Harrow to visit her husband, complained of feeling unwell and asked for an aspirin. Examination showed her to have a high temperature and an obvious yellow tint. The original discomfort she had felt in her upper abdomen in sympathy with her husband was, having subsided, being followed within five days by fever and developing jaundice.

Every surgery held by a local doctor now seemed to bring a fresh case into the open. The newly discovered sufferers, however, only confirmed Dr Kopelman's first impressions: the illness was confined almost entirely to adults. Among the first sixty cases, only six were in their teens. Time after time the victims presented themselves in pairs: a husband and wife, sometimes a mother and daughter, falling ill within hours of each other. The disease still showed a predilection for the more prosperous homes in the neighbourhood, and day after day Dr Kopelman found himself examining executives, teachers, doctors, solicitors, and their families, all displaying the distinctive lemon-coloured skin of early jaundice.

Every case presented Dr Kopelman with a diagnostic dilemma. An obscure jaundice can take a long time to disentangle, and all other possible causes had to be considered before any diagnosis of Epping jaundice could be made. (One unfortunate patient, who might at first sight have been mistaken for yet another victim, was found to have a slowly developing cancer blocking the bile ducts.) Even after a diagnosis of Epping jaundice was certain, Dr Kopelman's task became no easier. All he could say was that it was a disease that had as yet no name, that its cause remained undiscovered, that its clinical course was uncharted and its eventual outcome conjectural.

With an accumulation of experience Dr Kopelman became able to recognize the different ways in which the disease might present itself, there seeming to be three main variations in the clinical picture. A majority of patients suffered from an acute form like the one the medical student experienced. In these there was a dramatic onset, with fever and severe pains in the upper abdomen persisting for twenty-four to thirty-six hours. The illness then apparently paused for four or five days with the patient feeling generally unwell before fever returned and the jaundice deepened. In others, usually a partner of one of the acute cases, the disease came in gentler guise, as with the medical student's wife. Here there was only a vague discomfort, followed four or five days later by an onset of jaundice and general malaise. In the very elderly there was yet another presentation, with an onset so insidious that the first the patient knew was the appearance of a deep, persistent jaundice. In each victim the jaundice provoked intense itching of the skin.

Dr Ash, in his epic task of questioning and cross-examination, was similarly intrigued by the clinical picture. Although the symptoms of Epping jaundice were totally unlike those of infectious hepatitis, he paused to reconsider whether a virus might be responsible. The patients seemed to him to be describing an illness which had two phases: a dramatic onset followed, after a distinct pause, by fever and jaundice. Such a double-phased pattern of illness is characteristic of several different virus infections, the fully developed picture of poliomyelitis being a typical example. The Epping jaundice might therefore be caused by a new, hitherto undescribed virus. Yet try as he would, Dr Ash was able to trace no route by which such a virus infection might have passed between those households affected. None of the afflicted couples knew each other; they had no mutual acquaintances who could have acted as symptomless carriers.

He wondered next whether the infection was carried by food – but there had been no shared meal, no social occasion, buffet or dinner where the sufferers mingled, no institution or organization where they could have eaten food prepared in the same kitchens. Even their groceries and general provision lists looked completely harmless. Among all the family foodstuffs, only the bread came from a common source: the local bakery – but bread has hardly ever been implicated as a carrier of infection, and hundreds of people without the slightest trace of jaundice were buying bread from the same shop.

Knowing he could not afford to ignore the remotest line of inquiry, Dr Ash even considered the possibility that here was an insect-borne disease, carried from person to person as malaria is carried by the female *Anopheles* mosquito. Yet it all seemed highly improbable. The patients lived miles apart, their houses were scrupulously clean and the month was February, a cold, wet and inhospitable time of year for insects.

X-rays and pathological tests confirmed that no patient was suffering from gallstones or gall-bladder disease. By now, however, liver samples obtained by biopsy were being studied not only by Dr Robertson, the hospital pathologist, but also by other experts at the Royal Free Hospital in London. At last one fact grew clear: Epping jaundice was being precipitated by inflammation of the liver. More startlingly, however, the samples all showed the same picture: an inflammation involving the liver cells and minute bile ducts like nothing ever before described. It was a unique form of liver damage, and no known infection, poison or even drug could have produced anything remotely comparable. So far as the experts were concerned, it was an entirely new clinical condition with nothing to suggest a cause.

Dr Robertson and Dr Kopelman searched step by step for the slightest evidence of infection. Twelve cases underwent tests for glandular fever and its virus; another thirteen had immunological studies for the rare undulant fever. The Virus Reference Laboratory at Colindale performed extensive studies on specimens, searching for any virus that might have invaded the body through the intestines; the Leptospirosis Reference Laboratory examined specimens of blood to exclude the uncommon form of jaundice spread by rats and known to hygiene officers as 'ratcatchers' yellows', to doctors as Weil's disease; the Hospital for Tropical Diseases took up a search for any evidence of invasion of the body by liver fluke. Every test proved negative.

Mr Sanders, the biochemist at St Margaret's, tucked away, as he described it, 'safe in his cubby-hole', was contemplating the biochemical findings with fascination. He was beginning to form the view that these results could only be explained by a type of toxic injury to the liver caused by some chemical or drug, but the clinical findings under his scrutiny were those from the young anaesthetist, the wife of Dr Kopelman's assistant. The most superficial consideration of her work produced a monumental catalogue of drugs, gases and anaesthetic agents to which she might have been exposed.

Dr Ash was meanwhile putting together a list of the substances he would expect to find in any prosperous home, which had only recently been introduced on to the market and whose use was confined to adults. Inevitably his list began with the newly introduced contraceptive pill; but half the sufferers were men. Various forms of alcohol or tobacco likewise seemed excluded: abstainers and non-smokers were among the victims. He asked about illnesses and the consumption of tablets, searching for any new drug which might have been prescribed by a doctor or bought direct from a chemist. He emerged from his inquiries with a dossier of confusing, random information in which nothing made a connection.

Harry Kopelman's thoughts kept straying back to the start of the epidemic as he had seen it and the fact that the medical student's wife developed her first symptoms without leaving Harrow. Whatever caused her illness, germ or chemical, drug or toxin, her husband must have carried it to her from Epping. Close questioning, however, produced only the most unpromising answer. Before travelling home that day, the medical student purchased nothing more exceptional than a loaf of wholemeal bread.

Rumour was meanwhile abroad and working up for a storm. Others besides the medics concerned were beginning to realize that something unusual had happened. On Sunday, 21 February, the medical registrar at St Margaret's found himself facing a patients' insurrection. Several women in the later stages of pregnancy, admitted for treatment for raised blood pressure, were demanding to discharge themselves, regardless of any hazard to themselves or their unborn babies from leaving their blood pressures untreated. The chance of infection from jaundice became their greater anxiety. Gently and authoritatively the registrar restored order, pointing out that neither he nor any of the nursing staff handling jaundiced patients had shown the faintest sign of turning yellow. His reasonableness won the day.

Next morning, when the registrar went to give a brief report of the disturbance in the wards to Dr Kopelman and to recount the arguments used to restore peace, the doctor heard him out in silence. Then he quietly conveyed the news which had just reached him: one of their nursing sisters was being brought into hospital with what sounded like all the symptoms typical of Epping jaundice.

Harry Kopelman felt a degree of trepidation as he went to see the nursing sister after her arrival. The undertones of tension were reminiscent of a difficult oral interview in a medical finals exam on which something immensely important depends. Could this perhaps be the first instance of a person infected by contact with a known case? Was the sister only the first of a second generation of cases, the start of a second wave in the epidemic? Such a patient must surely hold the key to the mystery, if only he could sift it out.

With outward calm, Dr Kopelman began his consultation by noting a careful, systematic history, discussing everyone the sister had met, every case she had nursed, every place she had been in, everything she had done, every tablet taken, every food item consumed. Then, as she went over everything in her daily diet, almost casually she mentioned how a day or so before the onset she had bought a loaf of brown wholemeal bread. Dr Kopelman paused, stethoscope in hand.

There were at that point six patients suffering from Epping jaundice in the two medical wards of St Margaret's Hospital, and losing not a moment, Dr Kopelman made his way to each in turn. The first he questioned, a young foreign woman, the wife of an air force sergeant, was certain she had eaten nothing but white bread, bought 'ready cut'. All the other five, however, positively remembered eating this very type of wholemeal bread. Even as he began to reflect on the information, Dr Kopelman was interrupted by a staff nurse dashing after him from the female ward. The sergeant's wife had suddenly remembered how she had indeed purchased a loaf of wholemeal bread a day or so before falling ill.

Dr Kopelman's phone call to Dr Ash could not have been

made at a more timely moment. Pressures from mounting public concern were growing. Every councillor on the Epping and Ongar Rural District Council was becoming aware that the district was being swept by an epidemic, and it could only be a matter of days before the news broke in the press. Already the Health Department was the target for a barrage of anxious questions.

Armed with Dr Kopelman's discovery, Dr Ash set out to revisit as many sufferers as possible. Of the twenty-four patients he managed to question within the next few hours, twenty-three readily agreed they had bought and eaten the brand of coarse brown bread. In the end, practically every known sufferer from Epping jaundice recalled having eaten some of it, while one patient, a doctor, even remembered feeding a few crusts to his dog, admitting with surprise that the animal subsequently turned yellow. With commendable thoroughness the Pathology Department at St Margaret's Hospital set out to take a blood specimen from the dog, but unfortunately omitted the simple step of obtaining the animal's consent. In a brief but dramatic encounter only the dog succeeded in drawing blood.

Isidore Ash had already noted and been puzzled over the way the epidemic was distributed around two separate centres: the town of Epping and the village of Chipping Ongar, seven miles east. He was especially baffled by one elderly Ongar lady who, alone among all the patients, insisted she could not have eaten the wholemeal bread sold by the Epping bakery. It had been several years since she had ever travelled into Epping, she said. Dr Ash visited her three or four times to check and recheck her story, but her testimony remained unshakeable. On the last occasion her daughter arrived at the house just in time to overhear the repeated interrogation. But, she asked, hadn't her mother bought just such a loaf from the baker's in the village? It emerged that this was a newly opened branch of the Epping bakery concerned.

The main bakery stood in Epping High Street, a tidy establishment pervaded by the comforting smell of fresh-baked bread. Dr Ash, arriving unheralded, had his inquiries met with an alarmed courtesy but no lack of co-operation. Two things at once became apparent. First, the bakery was clean and hygienic, well organized and carefully run. Second, the manager was not available for questioning. Both he and his wife, it was said, were down with jaundice. In fact, Dr Ash was informed, the manager had just undergone a liver biopsy under Dr Kopelman's supervision.

Dr Ash was shown a loaf of the wholemeal bread. It was a rather specialized type, a coarse brown loaf with a distinctive texture and flavour. Children seldom cared for it, and it was, if anything, a bread for the connoisseur. Also, as the shop explained, it was an expensive bread. Suddenly Dr Ash saw why the Epping jaundice occurred on the whole in prosperous households.

This particular bread was baked on only three days a week, usually in batches of nine loaves: a total production of twenty-seven loaves a week. Dr Ash viewed the large metal bins where the wholemeal flour was stored, the mechanical dough mixer with its two rotating arms, the racks where the rising dough, neatly divided into bread tins, was left to stand, and finally the baking ovens. As he moved on his conducted tour, Dr Ash's sharp eye could spot nothing in the least irregular or potentially harmful. Their routines seemed impeccable. Nevertheless, the evidence was overwhelming. Beyond all reasonable doubt this particular bread was somehow the culprit, and Dr Ash prohibited its further production and sale.

Some sort of chemical poisoning was increasingly

becoming the most likely explanation, but, if so, what was the substance and how did it get into the bread? Dr Ash interviewed one man who had tasted a slice but spat it out, saying it tasted bitter and unpleasant. He had remained completely well. On the other hand, no sufferer from Epping jaundice expressed any complaints about it at all. The bread had been made and sold by the Epping bakery over a number of years with never a discontented customer. As he pieced the jigsaw together, Dr Ash was able to show how the very first patient with Epping jaundice fell ill on 1 February. The number of fresh cases occurring each day then rose quite rapidly, the greatest number appearing between 4 and 10 February. Now, by the end of the third week of February, when it seemed the incidence of new cases could well be diminishing, Dr Ash made two deductions. First, if something was going awry in the process of preparation and baking, it must have begun to happen in the closing days of January 1965. Indeed, if adulteration or contamination had been taking place, it must still be occurring, for fresh cases of Epping jaundice were still being diagnosed. Second, whatever substance was responsible acted very quickly and was remarkably toxic to the liver.

The bread was an unleavened bread made from only three constituents: wholemeal flour, salt and water. The same salt and water were used in the preparation of practically every item produced by the bakery, and all these were completely harmless. The one distinguishing feature of the coarse brown bread was its special ingredient: a specific wholemeal flour. Dr Ash inspected the flour again, but still could find nothing abnormal. Samples of flour taken from the half-empty storage bins were sent, together with unsold loaves, to the public analyst at Epping and the National Toxicology Laboratory at Carshalton.

Isidore Ash settled down to investigate detergents and cleaning agents used to clean and scour the bakery and its equipment. He asked about chemical poisons for killing and repelling the insects inevitably attracted by the warmth and abundant food of a bakery. He examined the lubrication of any machinery, to be sure the dough was not being contaminated by oil. He even surreptitiously investigated the mental state of the bakery staff in case one of them had accidentally or even maliciously sabotaged the process. There was nothing suspicious to discover.

On Tuesday, 2 March, Dr Ash issued a special report on the epidemic, and, realizing that his words would be widely reported, decided after much deliberation not to mention by name the precise item of food implicated. A week had gone by since he had prohibited the production and sale of the wholemeal bread. On the following Friday, 5 March, the *Epping Express and Independent* carried a twelve-inch headline across its front page: 'Mystery Illness Strikes, Local Food Suspect in Epping Outbreak; 60 Cases Reported'.

It was about now that an interesting fact emerged. The wholemeal flour used for the bread was ordered a sackful at a time, one sack, containing 140 pounds of flour, being enough to last the bakery for four to six weeks. The ordinary flour used in the white bread was delivered in routine bulk order by the miller's own lorry; the wholemeal flour, ordered a sackful at a time, came by special delivery. The last delivery of specialized flour had arrived in Epping on 21 January. It had then been stored in its sack, since the baker held almost a week's supply in hand. The baker was in fact quite certain that the last measure of the old was not used up until Saturday, 30 January. Only in the early hours of Monday, 1 February, was the new sack of flour tipped into the storage bins and the first scoopfuls taken for baking. Dr Ash promptly sharpened his focus on that one sackful of flour as a prime suspect.

All the wheat was ground at a mill in London in the same way, no matter for what purpose the flour was destined. The great bulk of the flour thus produced was dispatched directly to various bakeries. For the specialized type of wholemeal flour, however, bran was mixed back into the flour after grinding. This wholemeal mixture was then sent to another company so that various chemicals to make the flour rise could be added, and finally it was passed to a firm of distributors, who sold it to bakeries all over the country under a trade name. With a sense of relief Dr Ash could at least pass the task of inspecting the mill and the premises of the subsidiary firms over to the public-health teams of the London County Council.

Since the wholemeal flour was distributed throughout the country, it seemed worth checking to see whether similar outbreaks of jaundice were happening elsewhere. For the first time in his investigations, Dr Ash now ran into outright obstruction, the Ministry of Health pointedly refusing to issue a circular to other health departments. Surprised but unabashed, Dr Ash promptly drafted and circulated his own letter of inquiry.

On Friday, 12 March, the *Epping Express and Independent* was returning to the topic of the epidemic: 'Mystery Illness: Food Is Involved'. It was a brief column, desperately short of hard facts. It did no more than emphasize that the problem posed by Epping jaundice remained unsolved: 'Dr Ash, the town's Medical Officer of Health, said yesterday . . . , "There is no doubt that the food suspected of the outbreak is definitely involved. How it became contaminated remains a mystery." '

Four days later, on Tuesday, 16 March, the Epping and Ongar Health Committee listened uneasily and incommunicado to Dr Ash's interim report. The medical officer's position was fraught with difficulty. It was essential for the health committee, a meeting composed of anxious and concerned councillors, to be kept informed, but Dr Ash had precious little to offer beyond a series of guesses. There was no solid proof to support his analysis. The Epping jaundice could well become the subject of legal proceedings, yet he had to name the companies and products which he believed to be implicated while lacking the evidence to substantiate any allegations. He needed to avoid a statement which could provoke public alarm or panic, yet was also uncomfortably aware of being answerable for his handling of the crisis. The one hopeful aspect was that three weeks had passed since he prohibited the production and sale of the bread and no new cases had emerged for two weeks. Meanwhile most early victims seemed well on the road to recovery.

A few days later, the long-awaited analyst's reports on the bakery samples arrived. The results were frustratingly vague in implication. The public analyst, Dr J. Hammence, having performed a wide range of tests, could confidently exclude contamination of the unsold loaves by seeds of poisonous weeds, or by any alkaloid derived therefrom. He was also able to exclude any trace of metallic poisons or agricultural pesticides. In short, the loaves were completely harmless. On the other hand, the samples from the storage bin did show a minute trace of contamination: an infinitesimal amount of an organic base not normally present in wholemeal flour. With the techniques at the analyst's disposal it had been impossible to identify this chemical. It was present in a concentration of only thirteen parts in a million (0·0013 per cent). This must surely be virtually irrelevant, for how could so minute a quantity of anything provoke an illness as sudden and severe as the Epping jaundice?

As if to compound his problems, Dr Ash now received the reports from the London health authorities. The mill and subsidiary firms which produced and marketed the wholemeal flour had been thoroughly investigated. Their premises and procedures were entirely satisfactory. And to becloud matters even further, each post brought replies to the circulated letter of inquiry. No other unusual cases of hepatitis or jaundice were being reported. Epping stood alone in its predicament.

News of the curious epidemic began to spread rapidly, attracting inquiries from further afield. A phone call from a man in south London, who had been on holiday with his wife at the east coast, told how they had broken their journey home to buy sausages and a loaf of brown bread in Epping. Both were now suffering from jaundice. Was it the Epping variety? Could sausages therefore be the suspect food? There was a rueful report from a teacher who lived in Chelmsford but taught in Epping. He usually ate sandwich lunches cut from a locally produced coarse brown bread, and he, too, was suffering from jaundice. There was, on the other hand, one brief moment when the harassed Dr Ash felt he had done some good. A woman living thirty miles away had eaten bread from Epping, was now jaundiced, in terrible pain and in hospital, and about to undergo an exploratory operation. Her husband, reading of the Epping epidemic, hesitantly made contact. By a series of hasty telephone calls Dr Ash managed to arrange an exchange of clinical information and avert unnecessary surgery.

Dr Kopelman had, in charting the evolution of a new disease, by this time accumulated a considerable fund of information on its clinical aspects. Patients seemed to recover steadily and spontaneously. In almost all cases the jaundice, with its intolerable itching, began to improve after a week or so, though it usually took four to six weeks for it to clear completely. In only one or two cases were the symptoms exceptionally severe and prolonged, but even here Dr Kopelman felt hopeful. The body seemed fully capable of repairing the damage inflicted on the liver and smaller bile ducts. Almost all the early victims were growing cheerfully convalescent.

For Dr Ash, however, the problem of the cause could not be left to rest. The clinical picture was undoubtedly one of a toxic injury, but how could such a microscopic contamination be responsible? Since the numbers of new cases declined rapidly after the middle of February, it seemed that, as the epidemic progressed, so the bread became less toxic. Had this contaminating chemical therefore been spread unevenly in the sack of flour? Was the most contaminated portion used up before samples were taken? But samples from the time when the epidemic was at its height were needed to test the idea, and none survived.

How, in any case, could some unidentified chemical have got into the wholemeal flour? And why did Epping receive the only contaminated sackful in the country? If the flour was contaminated neither at the mill nor at the distributors, nor even at the bakery, then only one probability remained: the contamination must have come about in transit.

Dr Ash returned tenaciously to his inquiries and the fact that the wholemeal flour was brought to Epping by van as a special delivery, the contract for this being held by a small haulage company which transported a wide variety of goods throughout East Anglia. The firm had been satisfactorily delivering wholemeal flour to the Epping bakery over a considerable period.

Yes, the company's manager readily agreed, other goods were carried at the same time as the flour. Various chemicals were transported since the company distributed supplies for a firm of commercial chemists. Many different substances were carried by the hauliers, and it would be almost impossible to say precisely what chemicals, if any, might have travelled in the same van as the suspect sackful of flour. There had been no record of any spillage or damage to a chemical container on the date Dr Ash was specifying.

Dr Ash telephoned the equally mystified haulage firm several times, speaking on each occasion to the manager. At last he asked to talk directly to the van driver. The man was rarely in the office, but eventually a message came through that the driver did indeed remember a plastic chemical container having tipped up in the van at some point. The metal cap came off and a quantity of liquid was spilt among the other goods. He had no idea of what was in the container. Perhaps a gallon of liquid had been spilt in all. A number of parcels were damaged. Two or three packages wrapped in paper and obviously wet had been returned to the sender, but the driver felt sure none of the liquid had affected a sack of flour.

Dr Ash was by this time on the receiving end of unremitting pressure, both from the council chamber and the press. On 11 April, at a meeting of the Epping and Ongar Urban District Council, concern was shown over the persistent lack of information. One councillor, Mr Clark, urged his fellow councillors to press Dr Ash for as early a statement as possible. Another, Councillor Coster, feared some patients might have suffered irreparable damage. The clerk to the council promised that a report would be presented at the next meeting of the Public Health Committee, and on 16 April the *Epping Express and Independent* carried a column under the headline:

'Concern over Mystery Illness'. A certain criticism of the medical officer was implied if not directly stated.

The fact that the Epping jaundice was caused by eating brown bread from a high-street bakery was by now widely known. Dr Ash had feared the knowledge might provoke public alarm. It led instead to a welcome telephone call from an elderly lady to say she had bought brown wholemeal bread when the epidemic was at its height. She had thought it tasted bitter and threw it out for the birds, but not even the birds could be persuaded to eat it. It was still lying untouched in the middle of her lawn if they cared to come and collect it.

The retrieved sample consisted of two rather small pieces of rain-sodden bread which had lain in the open for several weeks. Dr Ash reflected ruefully that if the contaminating chemical was water-soluble, every trace must by now be washed out. Carefully, however, he divided the sample into equal parts, entrusting one half to the hospital laboratory and sending the other for analysis to the National Toxicology Laboratory at Carshalton, Surrey.

At St Margaret's the pathologist, Dr Robertson, venturing into unfamiliar territory, decided to carry out his own biological trials. He chose six young male white mice for his tests, feeding them on the brown bread and water. For comparison, he fed two other mice with white bread and water. The trial lasted ten days, and its results were conclusive. All the mice fed on the brown bread suffered liver damage. Microscopic examination moreover showed how the pathological changes in their liver tissues matched those in the liver biopsies of the human patients. The mice fed upon white bread meanwhile suffered no liver damage whatsoever.

Dr Robertson's chemical analyses were equally illuminating. He discovered the same unfamiliar organic chemical in the sample of bread as had been traced in the wholemeal flour, but this time it was present in considerable quantities. The concentration was 200 times greater than in the samples examined earlier. The contaminating substance in the bread retrieved from the lawn constituted 0·26 per cent of the bread, a finding confirmed by the Toxicology Laboratory at Carshalton. After a process of extraction, a yellow deposit remained, and here was the contaminating chemical in its pure form. Unfortunately, it was still too small an amount for the analytical techniques of the day to identify. Certain of its properties, however, could be discovered. If the deposit was suspended in alcohol and fed to mice, the characteristic liver damage occurred.

Dr Ash, armed at last with indisputable evidence, returned to the fray. It was customary, he found, for the haulage contractors to hold supplies from the chemical firm for several days in a warehouse before sending them on by road. The container which spilt could well have left the chemical firm two weeks before being upset in the van. With a longer time period to consider, and hence a longer list of items to choose from in addition to the technical information gleaned from the chemical analysis, the chemical firm was at last able to make a suggestion. The liquid involved in the spillage could well have been an epoxy-resin hardener, a bonding substance. This consisted of an aromatic ammonia derivative or amine which, when crystallized from benzene, consisted of pale yellow crystals. As a free base it was almost insoluble in water, though it dissolved readily in a trace of acid. The company willingly supplied samples of the amine as well as a dossier of all known information.

A series of comparative laboratory studies now placed the matter beyond dispute. The amine in the bonding liquid and the substance isolated from the sample of brown bread were identical. Every property matched. Epping jaundice was the

result of accidental poisoning by an aromatic amine technically known as 4,4'-diaminodiphenylmethane.

The amine possessed one rather unusual property. It slowly
darkened when exposed to sunlight. At long last Dr Ash
could reconstruct the sequence of events. The bonding liquid,
gradually darkening from pale yellow to brown, would not be
noticeable against the hessian of the sack or the rich brown
of the wholemeal flour. The sack then stood for several days
in the warm bakery, and by the time the staff came to handle
it the cloth was dry, the stain unnoticeable. When the sack
was tipped into the storage bin, the most heavily contaminated flour at the bottom came out on top, thus being the first
to be used and thus beginning the epidemic with precipitate
effect. By the time Dr Ash took samples from the half-empty
bin almost all the contaminated flour was used and gone.

About ninety loaves had been produced from the contaminated flour, but these were usually sold in quartered sections,
making in all about 360 portions of adulterated bread. Many
customers had bought more than one portion, and cases must
have occurred which were too mild to come to a doctor's
attention. Dr Kopelman and Dr Ash had nevertheless gathered
together records for almost a hundred sufferers. From the
consequent data available it became possible to calculate that
about half a dozen slices would have produced liver damage
in anyone who ate them.

Later biochemical studies rounded off the story. The amine,
once swallowed, was absorbed from the intestine and carried
by the bloodstream to the liver. Here it was broken down into
three or four highly toxic metabolites which were excreted by
the liver cells into the bile ducts. The metabolites caused
intense irritation of the ducts and hence considerable pain.
Within hours the ducts were inflamed and obstructed, the
surrounding liver cells damaged. Jaundice therefore set in.

On Friday, 8 May, the *Epping Express and Independent* devoted a double front-page column to a public statement from the Medical Officer of Health for Epping. Meanwhile, in the Epping and Ongar Council Chamber, councillors were calling on the Rural District Councils Association to press for government regulations to control the use of food-carrying vehicles. On Tuesday, 18 May, the Public Health and General Purposes Committee insisted on still more information from the medical officer. 'Is it true', demanded Councillor Stanley Deacon, 'that there are still cases of jaundice in the town?' Yet again Dr Ash found himself defending his strategy. On Friday, 21 May, the *Epping Express and Independent* spoke openly of criticisms of the medical officer in the council chamber.

At length, at the end of May, the House of Commons took official notice of the Epping jaundice when Stan Newnes, Member of Parliament for Epping, called upon Kenneth Robinson, Minister of Health, to make a statement. The minister's reply was based directly on Dr Ash's report. On Monday, 5 July, the topic was again aired in the House as the member for Epping rose to ask the minister about the need for regulations prohibiting the transporting of food in the same vehicles as dangerous chemicals. The mystery of the missing student had grown into a question of national concern.

Despite all the statements made in the press, the local council chamber and Parliament, many people still failed to understand exactly what had happened. In Epping a rumour persisted that the high-street bakery had been infested with rats which carried the disease to the bread. For many months the shop's trade dropped away and takings fell by half. On Sunday, 28 August 1965, however, the story of the Epping jaundice was told in the pages of a national Sunday newspaper, the *Observer*. For the first time true public recognition was given to the remarkable achievement of the medical team concerned.

At St Margaret's Hospital the team itself, consisting of doctors Kopelman, Robertson, Sanders and Ash, began to assemble their carefully harvested information for a concise article in the *British Medical Journal*. This duly appeared on 26 February 1966. In the medical world it brought them an instant respect which must have been an especial source of satisfaction to Dr Ash, since he had taken the brunt of public criticism and demands for action. The article was, in fact, the first account of a new kind of poisoning caused by a chemical only recently introduced into a commercial process. As such it was a classic of its kind. The *Journal of the American Medical Association* saluted it as 'a splendid example of scientific expertise and close co-operation among a wide variety of disciplines . . . a magnificent instance of scientific detective work, one which no one would believe if it were described as a fictional "whodunit" '.

By now the epidemic had long since run its course. One after another the patients recovered. For some there was a residual intolerance to certain foods, prolonged periods of listlessness, ill-defined symptoms and vague ill-health – but eventually in every one of them a sense of well-being was re-established.

About a year after the epidemic subsided the pet dog which had suffered from jaundice developed a severe diabetes. This did not respond to treatment and the animal had to be destroyed. A thorough autopsy confirmed that every trace of Epping jaundice had disappeared from its body. The disease which made it ill had been caused by a chronic disorder of the pancreas, the liver showing only those changes which might be expected in diabetes. There was no evidence of any permanent damage that could have been laid at the door of amine poisoning.

The dog was the only sufferer from Epping jaundice ever to come to post-mortem examination.

Chapter 4

The Ghost Disease

'The *zona* blows, and as the wind touches the people – men, women and children – they become possessed by the spirit which is within the *zona* and start to shiver as if all had been poisoned by *nagliza* sorcery' – R. M. Berndt, *Oceania*, 23:40, September 1952.

New Guinea is after Greenland the largest island in the world. Barely a hundred miles to the north of Australia, it lies within ten degrees of the Equator, a great mountain range which rises out of tropic seas and is blanketed by almost impenetrable rain forest. The forest, hot and humid, swarming with life in its most extravagant and exotic forms, covers the island. It spreads from the flat, swampy, coastal plains, over the irregular foothills, up on to the high central plateau at 6,000 feet, and peters out only on the flanks of the great mountains, where the snow-covered peaks stand as high as 15,000 feet above the sea. The great central plateau is broken by wide, deep valleys and the gorges of fast-flowing rivers. Each valley, separated from its neighbours by high mountainous ridges, resistant forest and sheer distance, seems an isolated world sheltering its particular varieties of animals and plants. From the edges of the forest the land drops away in steep slopes covered four or five feet deep by kunai grass. Here and there throughout the forest of the central plateau, and on the slopes of the great hidden valleys,

lie the scattered settlements and tiny hamlets of the Melanesian Indians, little pockets of humanity divided off from each
other by geography, variations in customs and culture, but
most of all by barriers of language. In a land barely twice the
size of New Zealand, at least 450 different tongues are spoken.

Generations of voyagers landed on the New Guinea coasts,
but the difficulty of travelling through the rain forest and a
lurking virulent strain of malaria protected the interior from
exploration until the present century. It was in 1936 that a
prospector, Ted Eubanks, first made a trek into the eastern
highlands, searching for gold to the south-east of Mount
Michael. He found no gold, but instead encountered huge
pine forests and a remarkable native people. Time had stood
still in the great hidden valley of the Yani river where the
tribes he discovered were relics of the Stone Age. Eubanks
was the first Westerner they had met, and they knew nothing
of the outside world. They had never seen the sea, let alone
heard of it. Their social structure was so basic that they had
no collective name for themselves or their tribe. Even the
name Fore Indian, by which they eventually came to be
known, resulted from a misunderstanding. It was based on
the description they gave to a neighbouring people.

These tribal peoples were short in stature, and despite the
frequent rain and occasional cold of the uplands went almost
naked. With no knowledge of textiles, they wore skirts and
capes made from plaited bark. They greased their skins with
animal fat and the adult men wore an animal bone piercing
the septum of the nose. Feathers, seeds, shells, ringlets of
hair, bones, the entrails and testes of animals, even human
fingers were worn as ornaments. They worked neither clay
nor metals. Their only domestic animals were the dog and
the pig, which shared their huts. The pig was especially
important as a sign of wealth and standing and a young piglet

might be carried cradled with a human baby and even suckled at the same breast.

The men hunted, but these were mainly agricultural communities, the women using a rudimentary digging-stick to plant and harvest taro and the sweet-potato. In the villages, the men lived communally in a large, central, circular hut, the women and children in smaller low huts arranged about it. At about the age of seven, boys left their mothers and underwent a prolonged and painful initiation ceremony before joining the men. Later observers commented on an apparent undercurrent of antagonism between the sexes.

Towards strangers they were suspicious and aggressive. Their lives were overshadowed by fears of sorcery and witchcraft and their world was thickly populated by ghosts. There was raiding and warfare between villages and tribes, ritual killing, even cannibalism of the dead.

In 1949, Papua New Guinea became Trust Territories of Australia. To help pacify the tribes of the interior and take the first steps in establishing an administration, the Australian government set up a series of patrol posts throughout the territories. In 1952, the first post in the area of the Fore Indians was established at Tarabo, one of the larger villages where a Lutheran mission had been founded three years earlier. It was a seldom-visited outpost from which 30,000 Melanesian natives were to be administered, policed and censused. The patrol officer and the missionary were the only Europeans in the entire region. Two years later the patrol post was moved a few miles east to the village of Okapa, which lay at the very centre of the Fore territories.

It was from the patrol officer in charge of this post, a young Australian, J. R. MacArthur, that first official reports came of an alarming phenomenon. On Sunday, 6 December 1953, he recorded in his patrol diary:

> Proceeding S.W. across range, and down and across a small creek ascending to Amusi villages, nearing one of these dwellings I observed a small girl sitting down beside a fire. She was shivering violently, and her head was jerking from side to side. I was told that she was the victim of sorcery, and would continue this shivering unable to eat until death claimed her within a few weeks.

Almost at once he was to realize that this was no isolated incident. Everywhere he went in the region, in every village, he came across women and children shivering and shaking until they sank into a slow paralysis and died. Everywhere he was given the same explanation. *Kuru*, the natives told him, with a tense insistence, was the result of sorcery.

In the Fore language, *kuru* means to shiver or tremble, as with cold or fear. It was the word given to a curious shivering and shaking which, anthropologists recorded, overtook certain tribes when the cold wind they called the *zona* or 'ghost wind' blew across the land. In its final meaning, it was also the name given to this strange bewitchment or curse that condemned its victim to a sure death.

There was a time-honoured ritual for inflicting kuru. A sorcerer had first to obtain, from whomever he intended to harm, some intimate particle or fragment such as rejected scraps of food, hair clippings, discarded clothing, ornaments or excreta. These particles, together with a crumbled stone and the leaves of certain plants, were bound in a bundle and tied with canes and vines. Beating the bundle with a stick, the sorcerer would call out his victim's name and recite a spell: 'I break the bones of your legs; I break the bones of your feet; I break the bones of your arms; I break the bones of your hands and finally I make you die.' Then he buried the bundle in muddy ground. As the bundle quivered and shook in the unstable, boggy morass, so the victim grew tremulous and unsteady. As the bundle rotted and disintegrated, so the sufferer's health gave way.

In August 1954, Patrol Officer MacArthur wrote: 'Kuru is definitely practised, but it must surely be psychological. I have sent some offenders (sorcerers) to Kainantu.' In certain regions, kuru was accounting for over half the deaths among women. There were villages where it was coming close to wiping out the population.

Slowly a fuller picture of the affliction emerged, both of its clinical details and of the beliefs which its sufferers attached to it. The onset was nearly always insidious, and it usually began with some minor disorder of gait or balance, perhaps as a woman was negotiating an obstacle such as the palisade fences between the kitchen gardens or a single-log bridge over a stream. These disturbances of movement became more conspicuous when the victim was tired and fatigued, maybe at the end of the day, or when she was still weak, recovering from fever or recent childbirth. A sharp eye might recognize a disturbance of gait at an early stage, simply from an odd but characteristic disruption in the swinging rhythm of a plaited-bark skirt. Sometimes the woman herself first became aware of her clumsy movements, complaining of unsteadiness and insecurity in her legs, a sensation the Fore Indians called 'loose knees'. More often she remained oblivious to the disorder until the dreadful day when its symptoms were pointed out to her by her husband or a relative.

The knowledge could be hard to bear. The unhappy woman now often became secretive and uncommunicative, trying to withdraw from the community, even retreating to a remote part of the forest. Inquisitive strangers were shunned and treated with anger and hostility. To everyone, but most of all to herself, she would deny that this was kuru, attributing loss of balance to arthritis or an old wound or scar. She would be troubled with headaches and leg pains, and suffer episodes of sheer terror. At times she would be racked by paranoid suspicions. Her well-being had been stolen away; she had been treacherously struck down by someone who knew her, by someone who had become her most deadly enemy, and she did not know who they were.

It was essential now to discover the sorcerer. If he could be unmasked, the damage might be mended, the danger averted. Husband and kinsfolk joined in a groping ritual hunt for the magician in which they perhaps collected water from numerous springs. If water from one particular spring caused her to retch violently or vomit, it was a sign that the bundle that was the kuru curse had been buried close by. A constant watch could now be kept on the spring, so that should the sorcerer come to inspect his curse or turn it in the ground he would be identified.

Alternatively, the victim's relatives might place clippings from her hair in one hollow bamboo tube and seal fresh-killed possum meat in another. The name of a suspected sorcerer would then be called aloud as the tubes were struck together and the one containing possum meat placed in a fire. Should the possum meat fail to cook, it was a sign that the suspect's name had altered the natural sequence of events and provided irrefutable evidence of guilt. Should a group, perhaps from a neighbouring village, be thought to harbour an unsuspected sorcerer, it might, as if from a goodwill gesture, be invited to share a common meal. Should one of the guests then fall ill after his return home, it was believed that he stood accused by the ghost of his still-living victim.

Where a sorcerer had been identified by one of these means, bribery might be tried to make him lift his curse.

More usually, however, husband and relatives would resort to *tukabo* or ritual killing. The unhappy individual identified would be waylaid in some isolated place, usually by three or four assailants. His arms, thighs and loins would be pounded with heavy stones, his windpipe bitten through so he could not name his attackers, his genitalia crushed with stones and clubs. In the full ritual of *tukabo*, slivers of bamboo or thorn would be inserted in his armpits and groin, the entrance wounds then being sealed with sap from a tree.

Just occasionally a transient improvement or even an illusory spell of normality seemed to prove the effectiveness of these counter-magic techniques. As a rule, however, the disease progressed without remission, the failure then being attributed to two sorcerers working simultaneously. Within a matter of months, in any case, the victim's walk would be so erratic that attempts to deny her state became hopeless and she returned to her community.

It was rare for a grown youth or man to develop kuru, but those who did seemed to find it almost impossible to come to terms with it. They tended to grow silent and withdrawn, even refusing food and thus dying of starvation long before a full picture evolved. Occasionally there were suicides, like the youth who declared he was not going to die like the other kurus and threw himself into a river.

Women victims seemed, by contrast, capable eventually of finding an inner strength and accepting their fate with a quiet resignation as they battled as long as possible to continue with daily tasks and fulfilling obligations to children and families. It was the loss of physical balance which was the most dramatic symptom as the condition progressed. For a while, walking might still be possible with the help of primitive crutches, but later on it could only be managed with a friend supporting each arm. At length standing was impossible; and sitting difficult without support. Now a stake would be driven into the ground outside the hut door so the stricken woman could sit holding on to it. Inside the hut a loop of plaited rope was hung from the roof for her to grasp for support. She struggled on for a time, sitting at the door of her hut, being carried to participate in pig-feasts and other social events. Soon even this became impossible. No longer able to lift herself from the ground, she was effectively bed-ridden.

Her family would still carry her from the hut to empty her bladder or bowels, but the most advanced symptoms nevertheless came on with dreadful speed. Her arms and legs grew so weak it was impossible for her to move them or feed herself. Her voice, at first becoming slurred, then disappeared, leaving her totally mute. With swallowing difficult, she choked on her food. Finally there was double incontinence and family or friends no longer carried her into the sun, but left her to lie untended in the hut's dark recesses. Mercifully, death came at last, perhaps from starvation, from septicaemia, from bronchopneumonia, from great pressure sores, or even from burns caused by falling on to the fire that burnt in the middle of the hut floor. By the time death claimed her, scarcely eighteen months to two years would have gone by since the first wavering symptom.

Serious medical attention began to be paid to kuru in 1955 when another patrol officer sent a typical kuru victim the twenty-five miles to Kainantu where the Government District Medical Officer, Dr Vincent Zigas, examined the woman and kept her under observation. His first suspicion agreed with the patrol officer's that here was a case of hysteria. Within a few months, however, after studying more and more cases, he found himself driven to an inescapable conclusion: kuru was no psychological phenomenon but some rare organic disease that matched nothing in his experience. Among the Fore Indians there existed a disease so rare, so unique, that it had managed to remain undescribed in 2,500 years of records. As far as he could tell, it appeared nowhere else on earth, yet here among these people it was occurring not as a few isolated cases but as a massive epidemic.

In the autumn of 1956, Dr Zigas put everything else aside and moved to Okapa. For several weeks he studied victims of kuru, marshalling every clinical technique at his command. Blood tests, virus studies and tissue specimens, taken from twenty-six sufferers, were flown to Melbourne in Australia for further investigation at the Walter and Eliza Hall Institute for Medical Research. Within weeks, Zigas knew he was defeated. The results were unhelpful: blood tests and chemical studies normal, attempts to grow viruses failing, investigations negative for all rare disorders known to occur in Papua New Guinea. Reluctantly Zigas recognized that the task was immense and he could accomplish nothing alone. He had no diagnosis, no clue even to the disease's nature.

The Walter and Eliza Hall Institute came under the direction of a distinguished medical scientist, Sir Frank Macfarlane Burnet. Both the institution and the trust territories administration were already aware that the problem of kuru was unlikely to be solved quickly. The prospect was rather for a long-drawn-out programme of field studies backed by laboratory research. It was at this point, in March 1957, that Zigas received an unexpected visitor to the Eastern Highlands District.

D. Carleton Gajdusek was a young American research scientist who already trailed a reputation for owning a brilliant intellect. He had been working as a visiting investigator on auto-immunity and the virology of infectious hepatitis under Macfarlane Burnet at Melbourne during the previous two years, but now, the appointment completed, was returning to Harvard to continue with his own project on child growth and development and disease patterns in primitive cultures. He had dropped off in New Guinea on his way home, in part to visit Macfarlane Burnet's son Ian, a patrol officer, and in part to take a look at kuru, his interest alerted by early reports. The disease could, after all, have some relevance for his paediatric studies.

The clinical descriptions of the disease were so bizarre that Gajdusek admitted he had read them with scepticism. Within two days of arriving at the Okapa patrol post he was seeing them for himself on every side. In people of all ages and both sexes, but mainly in women and children, he observed classical signs of progressive 'parkinsonism', terrible and relentless in their effects. As he wrote to a colleague in the United States:

> To see whole groups of well-nourished healthy young adults dancing about, with . . . tremors which look far more hysterical than organic, is a real sight. But to see them, however, regularly progress to neurological degeneration in three to six months (usually three) and to death is another matter and cannot be shrugged off.

Gajdusek was never a man to shrug anything off. Within days he had made his decision: he would join forces with Vincent Zigas to probe what was clearly some kind of degenerative disorder of the central nervous system, affecting a human population on a quite amazing scale. Within days he was learning the tribal language and compiling family histories of victims, in effect taking on his own shoulders a massive research project with no funding grants promised, no official backing from any government or academic institution. He was prepared, he said, to support it out of his own resources and to stick to it as long as he could, even should no outside funds become available.

Gajdusek was never a man, either, to wait on the niceties of official protocol, and he was under no illusions that he might be causing fluttering in administrative dovecots or creating feelings, back in Melbourne, that he was pre-empting others' research plans. 'Orthodoxy in intrusion into problems of medical investigation – in so far as ideas of others are not usurped without full acknowledgement – has never bothered me,' he wrote. 'The problem of medical investigation is an open field, and one which to me has always been noncompetitive.'

In early April he managed to ignore a telegram from the administration in Port Moresby asking him to stop work till the situation could be properly discussed. He wrote to Sir Macfarlane Burnet that he would like to remain until he had exhausted whatever he could contribute to the problem on the spot. Since they had selected paediatric material for special attention, he said, he doubted 'that there is anyone around or likely to be soon around who can complete these studies any better than I. I therefore consider it a duty both to the kuru patients and to my intellectual curiosity to stick to it for a month or longer as the matter works out.' He had established his claim as well as his right, if he so wished, to be seen as a controversial figure, and now it was perhaps a question of the administration accommodating itself to Gajdusek rather than the other way about. Macfarlane Burnet summed up his personal view of the whole sequence in a letter he wrote at the end of May:

Gajdusek really had no business in that field at all . . . But when he heard of the kuru situation, which we were arranging to investigate in a month's time, nothing could stop Gajdusek and in a week's time he had taken over the whole show and was working twenty hours a day as the self-appointed representative of the Hall Institute. Both the Administration and I were extremely annoyed for a week or two. However, I have a sort of exasperated affection for Gajdusek and a great admiration for his drive, courage and capacity for hard work. Also there is probably no one else anywhere with the combination of linguistic ability, anthropological interest, and medical training who could have tackled this problem so well. So everything is now in order; we are acting as a base for any laboratory work . . . and Gajdusek is being given full Administration support.

The Kuru Research Centre was established at Okapa, practically in the centre of the kuru region, and it featured as its hospital a large building constructed from native materials. To this were added a laboratory and examination room so that special examinations and clinical studies could be carried out on site. Specimens for more specialized studies were to be hurried by jeep along the rough track to Kainantu, twenty-five miles to the north, and from there flown by light aircraft to Port Moresby and on, by regular air service, to Australia or the United States.

At the hospital the doctors found they had patients 'walking in and deteriorating so rapidly and in so stereotyped a fashion that it is hardly believable'. Gajdusek was able to define kuru as 'a major, perhaps *the* major death threat, and cause of vendetta killings in the tribes today . . .' By July 1957, over 500 earlier deaths had been located and over a hundred patients had emerged, all dying. Gajdusek was in no doubt that they were dealing with a subject of fundamental importance, an illness which was causing over half the deaths in the race it affected. Whether it had a genetic, toxic or infectious origin, medical science was bound to have much to learn from it. He was already convinced that he was working in 'the best site in the world for study of chronic progressive degeneration' of the central nervous system. To solve kuru could hold out future hope for those who suffered from such degenerative disorders as parkinsonism, multiple sclerosis or even Huntington's chorea. By mid August, they knew of 150 active cases within a population of 15,000.

The sheer magnitude of the case loads was overwhelming, but Gajdusek and Zigas recognized quite rapidly how the clinical picture of kuru could vary. Children and adolescents suffered an especially rapid onslaught, the downhill progress proving more startling and precipitate than in the adult. In the elderly, the degenerative course was more protracted. For a long time before the onset of definite signs, minor symptoms might come and go, fluctuating from week to week and month to month. In elderly, chronic sufferers, however, dementia was often to the fore, confusion and disorientation setting in as the mind itself was destroyed.

The difficulties of compiling an accurate description of the disease were immense. It was often hard to understand what the Fore Indians meant by their descriptions of symptoms. Their belief that various disorders could be attributed to witchcraft or ghosts caused a certain confusion of terminology. It was also necessary to disentangle clinical findings which had nothing to do with kuru. Liver enlargement was found in about a third of kuru sufferers, but then, it turned out, liver enlargement existed in about a third of all Fore Indians examined, regardless of whether or not they had kuru. This symptom seemed more to be the result of the chronic endemic malaria.

Hence it was necessary to understand all other diseases and abnormalities which occurred in the area, and even what passed for normal among the Fore. There was, for instance, in one tribe a harmless tremor of the head and hands which appeared only in certain families. All the many investigations that faced Gajdusek or Zigas, their clinical examinations, blood tests, immunological studies and biochemical estimations, needed to be compared and contrasted with samples drawn from the general population before any accurate description of kuru could emerge.

Gajdusek had arrived in Papua New Guinea with one preconceived idea. He had fully expected to find that kuru was a form of meningo-encephalitis, an acute inflammation of the brain and its linings, caused by viruses. Now, in the field, he found nothing to support the theory, none of the rigors or heavy sweating of an acute infection, no change in the blood, no change in the cerebrospinal fluid from around the brain. Specimens sent to Australia and the United States failed to show any trace of a virus after several long weeks of animal culture. More important, there was no evidence for case-to-case transmission. Questioning failed to reveal anything to suggest that people who lived in close contact with a kuru sufferer for months at a time were any more likely to catch the disease.

Gajdusek reluctantly abandoned the idea of an acute infection and turned his attention to the fact that, on rare occasions, encephalitis may occur as a late complication of such virus infections as measles or mumps. Yet a search among kuru victims for consistent evidence of a preceding infection revealed nothing. Gajdusek and Zigas used their research centre as a general hospital, helping the Fore Indians through epidemics of mumps, measles, chicken-pox and whooping cough, besides outbreaks of bronchopneumonia and gastroenteritis among infants. They saw cases of bacterial meningitis and viral encephalitis, but never in association with kuru. New cases of kuru appeared every few days but never as a sequel to any other disease.

Accidental poisoning caused by an unrecognized toxic

substance in the environment was the next natural line of inquiry. Possibly an organic poison could be involved, while traces of heavy metals like mercury, zinc, manganese or copper are also known to cause a slow degeneration of the parts of the brain which co-ordinate movement and balance. An intensive study began of diet, of the soil where food was grown, of cooking methods, even of cooking-fire ashes. Any fungi, grubs and insects regarded as delicacies were investigated. Ashes used as 'salt' were analysed, as were the pigments with which the Fore decorated their bodies. Exhaustive checks were made for toxic substances in the blood, serum, urine, faeces and cerebrospinal fluid of kuru sufferers. Not a single finding emerged.

When the question of a vitamin or dietary deficiency was considered, the diet of the Fore Indian was found to be superior to that in many other New Guinea communities. It was reasonably varied with a high calorie content and a good quantity of protein. In any case, once sufferers from kuru were brought into hospital, they were fed on a full, controlled diet with no evidence of a remission.

Employing his encyclopedic memory and an unusual awareness of other disciplines, Gajdusek even turned for a moment to make a comparison with pasture syndromes, diseases that occur only in flocks feeding on pastures that are contaminated by minute quantities of a toxic substance or have a trace-element deficiency. Sheep that graze on Australian or New Zealand pastures where phalaris is the predominant grass, for example, develop a disorder similar to kuru known as the 'phalaris staggers' unless the deficiency is made up with frequent feeds of soluble cobalt salts. Gajdusek even considered complicated metabolic interactions in which excess of one chemical could lead to deficiency of another.

All these complex lines of reasoning were, in the end,

defeated by quite simple facts. Fore Indians who moved out of the region, even out of the interior, still developed kuru. One Fore Indian went to work on a plantation in the coastal plains, sharing the same diet of rice, tinned meat and other supplements as the other labourers. Nevertheless, after seven months, kuru made its first insidious appearance and then progressed to its fatal termination.

The failure to unravel the problem presented Gajdusek and Zigas with immediate practical concerns. Lacking any understanding of the disease, they could offer no rational treatment yet had a hospital full of deteriorating and dying cases. On a grim trial-and-error basis, they applied any treatment which might have the remotest chance of success. High dosages of sulphonamides and antibiotics were given to stamp out any concealed infection. Vitamin injections, cod-liver oil concentrates and crude liver extracts were administered to counteract the unlikely possibility that the disease was caused by a deficiency of a vitamin which had yet to be discovered. Since the central nervous system can be damaged by a shortage of cyanocobalamin and folic acid, these substances were given in almost excessive dosages. Steroids and antihistamines were prescribed to suppress any immunological reaction that might have escaped detection. Injections to remove traces of heavy-metal poisons from the body, even though none had been found, anticonvulsants, hormones, the humble aspirin itself were all tried, but time and again Gajdusek and Zigas nevertheless stood at the death-beds of patients, conducted hasty and distasteful post-mortems and laboured at endless series of studies.

The hopes of the Fore Indians had at first run high, their intense fear of kuru combining with the expectation that the doctors' magic could be stronger than their own. As they began to recognize medicine's ineffectiveness in the face of kuru, they helpfully suggested that the doctors might be proceeding along the wrong lines. If a camera photographed everyone in a village, would not the sorcerer's image appear in the photograph holding a kuru bundle; or could not the ophthalmoscope with which the doctors examined their patients' eyes be used to glimpse a sorcerer's rotting soul? They persisted with their own searches for remedies. A 'curer', preferably from a distant village, would lapse into a trance, often induced by drugs or the prolonged smoking of a bamboo pipe. In his trance he would gain, it was thought, access to hidden information and so identify the sorcerer. The kuru victim was meanwhile made a medicinal meal of pork, bespat with ginger and forest herbs, while for the heavy aching limbs there was a skin-pricking ritual with tiny arrows shot from a miniature bow.

Gajdusek knew that there had to be some extraordinary causative factor in the Fore Indians' lives or environment, if only he could recognize it. He compiled a long chronological table listing every known event in the history of the Fore, the introductions of new materials, the disappearances of old practices and customs. He listed everything which could conceivably be correlated with changes in the incidence of kuru. The table began at the start of the twentieth century and reached to the present; it started with the introduction of the sweet-potato and ended with the distribution of soap; it listed the last use of stone axes and included the eradication of yaws from the population by penicillin. He even included cannibalism, though cannibalism had been suppressed and kuru was increasing.

There were a few cases for which cures were claimed in individuals for whom native counter-sorcery seemed to have worked. Gajdusek found that some of these were where the earliest signs, precipitated by exhaustion or other illness, disappeared with a return of strength, the full ravages of kuru then inexorably reappearing in the course of time. Other supposed recoveries had been from episodes of hysteria where terrified girls mistook a mild or imagined symptom for a manifestation. The sad conclusion was that no individual who developed unequivocal kuru ever survived.

Investigating intensively, working almost night and day, Gajdusek nevertheless sought to preserve an overall view, trying not to lose himself in clinical minutiae or the quantities of suffering. Regarding the historical and geographical distribution of the disease, he asked how long it was since this strange epidemic first afflicted the Melanesians? How widely was it dispersed, and what boundaries had halted its spread? Accompanied by native orderlies and interpreters, he set out on a kuru safari, attempting to trace every case of kuru that had ever occurred. But in asking about the past there was an unexpected difficulty since the Fore Indians had no calendar. Being so close to the Equator meant there was little difference between the seasons: no summer and winter as such, only a rather vague and variable progression of dry and rainy seasons.

Yet while the Fore Indians had no conception of a year and a ludicrous inability to assess their own ages, their intelligences and memories were good. They could, for example, give reliable accounts of sequences of births within villages, placing individuals constantly and reliably in correct birth order. In each village Gajdusek would therefore line up the children in order of birth to form a visible, living calendar. Now it became possible to talk in such terms as 'before E was born' or 'a few days after C was born'. By relating this time-scale to his own assessment of children's ages and such known events as the date of the first government patrol into the area, he was able to plot events with reasonable accuracy.

Constantly cross-checking between these accounts, Gajdusek was able to extend his researches to cases occurring as many as thirty or forty years earlier. Everywhere he was told the same story: that in the past kuru was not a common disease, that it had only assumed its plague dimensions within living memory. The few really elderly surviving tribespeople insisted that this was so. Gajdusek found it hard to accept: so far as he could tell, the disease's incidence had been steady over the past few years. He reasoned that the old people's memories of cases occurring during their own childhoods must be unreliable since young children are often oblivious to the details of events happening in the adult world about them. Furthermore, from the anthropological viewpoint, surely any disease which had given rise to such an extensive system of beliefs and folklore must have been in a community for generations.

Within a few weeks, Gajdusek was able to produce maps showing that kuru was confined within an area roughly thirty-five miles long by twenty-five across, and that it had only been contained by definable geographical boundaries in the south-east, where it halted abruptly at the edge of the gorge of the Lamari River, and to the south-west, where it petered out on the margin of vast uninhabited tracts of rain forest. Elsewhere, where neighbouring peoples had resisted every social contact with the Fore, the disease halted abruptly. By contrast, where neighbouring people had a long history of social contact, trading, fighting and intermarrying with the Fore, kuru occurred in all their adjacent border villages. It was noticeably the Fore women who came as wives who brought the disease, spreading it first to their own children, then to more distant relatives.

Having travelled more than 1,000 miles on foot, spoken to thousands of witnesses and made a rough but impressive survey of an area almost 800 miles square, Gajdusek at last felt he could begin to discern a pattern to kuru: no European had contracted it; Fore Indians who had left their communities years before could develop it; Fore women spread it to neighbouring communities by passing it first to their children. Tentatively he went at last for the genetic option, advancing the hypothesis that kuru could be a familial or inherited disease.

Certain problems were at once apparent. Some rare degenerations of the central nervous system, like Huntington's chorea, are known to be genetically determined, but no other inherited disease has shown such a devastating incidence. While these diseases may afflict many members within a family, overall they remain quite rare in the community. Most awkwardly, however, some rather complicated theories of heredity became necessary to explain kuru's strange predilection for appearing in adult women and children. The genetic explanation did not sit as comfortably as Gajdusek would have wished, but he could find no other that came anywhere near to fitting the facts. The Fore Indians seemed fated to suffer their strange and dreadful epidemic.

Gajdusek decided the time had come to leave the field and return to the laboratories. He emerged from Papua New Guinea to find himself famous, the outside world fascinated. Medical journals were anxious to publish his papers on kuru; learned societies in the United States and Europe invited him to lecture. There was also a transitory barrage of curiosity from the press and general public, and the popular papers' especially inept and irritating dubbing of kuru as 'the laughing death' on the basis of a phrase taken out of context in a medical journal. Once the publicity died away, however, only the medical press continued the debate with academic speculations on the inheritance mechanism involved. In children, where the disease had an early onset, it seemed probable that the gene came from both parents, the child being in genetic terms homozygous. Where the onset of the disorder was delayed until adult life, it was thought the gene must be inherited from one parent only, the sufferer being heterozygous. Perhaps the gene needed certain hormonal circumstances for the disease to express itself, thus accounting for the preponderance of adult female victims.

In many Fore villages kuru had so depleted the female population that there was now a gross preponderance of men, as many as two or three to every woman. The men were therefore tending to leave their tribal lands to seek new lives and families in neighbouring or even distant communities. The administration began to fear they would take the kuru gene with them and so make the disease endemic over even greater areas of Papua New Guinea. By July 1960, the Australian government felt impelled to act and enacted the first genetic law in history, placing the Fore Indians in quarantine. No Fore would be allowed to leave the tribal territory and those who had left already must return.

In the Fore territories themselves circumstances were changing fast. The hospital at Okapa had become a permanent institution, staffed by the government medical services. With the help of patrol officers, teams of medical orderlies maintained the census and kuru records in every village. Anthropologists watched and studied the changing culture as nose ornaments were abandoned, traditional skirts and capes of plaited bark discarded for Western clothing. The initiation ceremonies for boys faded out, the men moved from the central, circular hut to live with their families in smaller huts, built now in a square-frame style and standing in neat rows. With the suppression of raiding and inter-village warfare, the structure became looser and more open. Here and there families decided to build a home in an isolated spot, separated from the main community.

The medical scientists were meanwhile finding it harder and harder to fit observations of kuru incidence into any statistical model based on a genetic assumption. Furthermore, there was the odd inconvenient occasion when a girl from a neighbouring tribe married into a Fore village and contracted the disease even though she had no Fore blood in her. The first hint of another possibility came in 1959 when W. J. Hadlow, a veterinary scientist, wrote an open letter to the *Lancet* in which he remarked on the resemblances between kuru in man and a disorder called scrapie recognized in sheep. Scrapie only occurred in sheep in certain flocks. It could appear in sheep introduced into the flock from outside and often struck down an animal months after it was removed from the flock. There were striking similarities in the pathological damage which each disease caused, but more importantly it had been found that if suspensions of brain tissue were taken from an animal which died from scrapie and injected into another, the second animal developed the disease about two and a half years later.

Gajdusek considered the suggestion with a dismayed reluctance. It made nonsense of the virus studies conducted at Okapa, when animal inoculation tests had been followed for only the customary few weeks. Now it was implied that months or even years might be necessary for a conclusive result. The prospect of having to repeat the studies was daunting enough, let alone the subsequent need to wait several years for the outcome. In any case, it sounded too much like another of the many blind alleys already patiently investigated.

Nevertheless, in the summer of 1962, Gajdusek returned to Okapa. Once again he set up his case studies, conducted post-mortems, froze and packed the brains removed from fresh kuru victims and hurried them to the airstrip for dispatch to the United States. Back in the laboratories of the National Institute of Neurological Diseases and Blindness, at Bethesda, Maryland, with specimens from seven known kuru fatalities he prepared suspensions from the brain tissue and injected them into chimpanzees. Curiosity and an intellectual honesty led him to repeat the experiment for all those degenerative diseases of the brain for which no cause was known. Then he settled down to the long, slow wait.

It was in late 1965 that the chimpanzees began to fall ill as, one by one, they developed a disease which appeared to carry all the marks of kuru. Fascinated and enlightened, Gajdusek filmed the stumbling, unsteady animals, repeated the clinical studies he had made at Okapa, and prepared to announce to the world that kuru had nothing to do with inheritance. It was, instead, a transmissible, infectious disease caused by a virus unlike any virus hitherto identified in man. Kuru was, in fact, the first disease known to affect *Homo sapiens* which could be attributed to infection by a 'slow virus', a virus that had an incredibly long incubation period. All the victims that he studied must have caught their illness years before he arrived in Papua New Guinea, but how had they caught it, and why was it only among the Fore that kuru spread as an epidemic? And why were the women and children so often struck down while the men for the most part escaped unharmed?

The answers came almost at once from two anthropologists, Robert and Shirley Glasse, who had repeated at leisure the surveys which Gajdusek conducted in haste and reinterpreted

his findings. Kuru was indeed, as the Fore Indians maintained, a relatively new disease. The first case seemed to have
occurred no longer than fifty years before in the village of
Uwami in the Keiagaua province of the North Fore. It then
gradually spread from village to village, reaching Paiti in the
south-west of the region as recently as 1950. The Glasses had
one further dramatic point to make: the spread of kuru was
inextricably linked with cannibalism.

While cannibalism had been usual among other tribes in
Papua New Guinea, it was a relatively new practice among
the Fore. It began in about 1915, when Fore Indians visiting
hamlets in the north among the Kamano peoples observed
the practice, were invited to participate, tasted human flesh,
liked it and took their new enthusiasm home. With remarkable speed, it then ceased to be a gastronomic matter and
became an accepted and important part of funeral ritual.
Custom demanded that the body first be left three or four
days to putrefy before being baked. Every part of the body
was then consumed, and there was a strict division of parts
between different relatives. By custom, the mother's brother's
wife had first claim to the brain. After the meal, remnants of
unconsumed fat were rubbed into the skin.

There were two important incidental factors. The first was
that it was difficult to sterilize food by cooking at that
elevation in the highlands where water boiled at a temperature of 95°C, and hence the human meat must always have
been underdone. The second concerned the identity of
partakers in the feast, diners consisting as a rule only of adult
women relatives and their children. The men usually
declined, fearing that such a meal might impair their fighting
ability.

The idea that cannibalism could be involved was not a new
one. From the beginning, patrol officers and other Europeans

had speculated that it might be so; the basic problem was that no one could see how. Gajdusek himself had wondered whether there might be a link. With the arrival of missionaries and police patrols, cannibalism had been discouraged and suppressed, though Gajdusek had sometimes suspected that an illicit cannibal ritual was being held. He found it impossible to believe, however, that all the many victims of kuru he observed could be partaking in forbidden feasts.

The picture was clear at last: kuru was caused by a transmissible, virus-like agent being conveyed by mouth from person to person as the mortal remains of sufferers were consumed by their relatives. Anything between two and twenty years could then intervene before the disease became apparent. His adult cases had contracted kuru before even the missionaries arrived in the Fore territories.

For the first time Gajdusek saw a glimmer of hope for the Fore Indians. With cannibalism suppressed, kuru would surely die out progressively. Those cases with the shortest incubation period, the violent cases in young children, would disappear first; those with a more prolonged incubation period, the adolescents, would disappear next; and last of all, the very slow onset cases would finally vanish from the community.

As Gajdusek worked in his laboratories, a second triumph came to his team when another group of chimpanzees fell ill. These had been inoculated with material from cases of Creutzfeld–Jacob disease, a rare sporadic disorder that occurs throughout the world as a premature senility in individuals still in the prime of life. This was the second slow virus disease to be recognized in man.

The studies at Bethesda threw a remarkable light on the viruses of both kuru and Creutzfeld–Jacob disease. They were smaller than any previously known viruses, and, although their size could be measured by filters, they remained invisible under the electron microscope. Gajdusek suspected them of being more closely related to viroids, a group of viruses known to occur in plants, consisting of nothing more than tiny fragments of genetically active material. Distinguishing between the viruses in the laboratory in fact presented a great difficulty. When a sporadic case of Creutzfeld–Jacob disease turned up in a tribesman from one of the other tribes of the interior, Gajdusek hazarded a guess. Perhaps it had originally been a sporadic case of Creutzfeld–Jacob dementia which occurred among the Fore Indians and was consumed. The virus, then passing from sufferer to sufferer by cannibalism, could easily have altered its clinical presentation to become kuru.

This could only ever be speculation, but there were certain more immediate and alarming implications. If slow-virus disease could be transmitted from individual to individual by the inoculation of tissue suspensions, then every patient who received a form of transplant was at risk. The fear was confirmed in 1974 when it was recognized that Creutzfeld–Jacob disease had been transmitted between two individuals by corneal transplant, the disease appearing eighteen months after the operation. Soon reports followed of a neurosurgeon who had died from Creutzfeld–Jacob disease after operating on the brain of a sufferer.

Gajdusek found himself drawing up rules and codes of conduct to protect both patients and surgeons in future transplant operations. He had said back in the early phases of kuru investigation, having dropped in on them more or less by accident, that he could not accept the phenomenon as 'a minor problem of a stone-age people. It is more than that, and if solved will certainly give to medicine important new leads.' This prophecy was fulfilled, and in 1976 he received the Nobel Prize in medicine for his work on the origin and spread of infectious diseases and as a recognition of the role he had played in that fulfilment. His other prophecy was also fulfilled as, year by year, the epidemic died out from among the Fore Indians and kuru came to be consigned to history.

Chapter 5

Death in the Parish

In 1817 rumours of a new disease came out of India. Asiatic cholera, as this pestilence came to be called, was not only killing thousands but advancing through every population that stood in its path. In a slow but irresistible tide, the disease burst out of the Indian sub-continent, spreading from country to country until, in 1831, in spite of every precaution it crept into the United Kingdom through the port of Sunderland. By the spring of 1832 it was rife in London and over 7,000 of the inhabitants died. Then, early in 1833, without visible reason, the epidemic burnt itself out and the disease disappeared. It was a brief respite. Fifteen years later, in 1848, Asiatic cholera returned but this time Afghanistan was its cradle and it slipped into Britain by way of London, spreading out through towns and cities in a nation-wide epidemic which was not extinguished until the final months of 1849. In London, nearly 7,000 people had died in a single month.

The inhabitants of the prosperous but overcrowded parish of St James, Westminster, however, congratulated themselves on escaping relatively lightly in each epidemic. In 1831–2 they suffered only thirteen deaths per 10,000 of the population, and in 1848–9 only fifteen deaths per 10,000, the mortality figures for London as a whole having stood respectively at fifty-six and seventy-six deaths per 10,000. Not even the clergy considered attributing this fortunate escape to a divine intervention. By the more up to date and scientifically minded it was thought to be owed to Farr's principle of elevation. During the 1848–9 epidemic, William Farr, the statistician at the office of the Registrar-General, analysing the registration of cholera deaths parish by parish, had observed a remarkable correlation. In London cholera mortality was related to the height of a district above the Thames: the greater the altitude, the fewer the deaths that occurred. Elevation, it seemed, conferred a relative immunity, and the parish of St James was placed a salubrious sixty feet above the Trinity high-water mark.

Mr Farr's principle of elevation was at the time one of the few 'certainties' concerning cholera. The subject had been extensively investigated, but the cause of the disease and the factors which precipitated an epidemic remained a total mystery. Attempts were made to relate outbreaks to such varying factors as rainfall, air temperature, changes in wind force and direction, the temperature of the Thames, even the presence of ozone and 'electricity' in the atmosphere. The number of suggestions far outstretched the known facts.

The theory favoured by the medical profession was that in certain circumstances, in the presence of filth, gross overcrowding, foul smells emanating from bad drains, and stagnant or stale water, a process of fermentation could be set in motion which produced a poisonous miasma. This miasma, when inhaled, then caused cholera. Since not everybody exposed caught the illness, it was felt that certain people developed a constitutional predisposition. Several different factors, including the use of hard or impure water, were thought to contribute to such a predisposition, but basically a cholera epidemic was considered to be the result of widespread air-borne poisoning.

The first intimations of a third epidemic came in 1853. Cholera had never quite died out in Poland and Eastern Europe, and already it was in the Baltic ports. During the first week in July, the chief mate of a vessel from the Baltic Fleet arrived home with the soiled linen of a sick officer. Within days, Asiatic cholera was diagnosed in London, and two months later Newcastle was in the throes of its worst outbreak, the death-roll reaching 1,500.

An epidemic on the grand scale looked inevitable, but in London the threat hung fire. Throughout the closing months of 1853 and the early ones of 1854, a few sporadic cases occurred. In April there were four deaths, in May four more, in June only three. Then, in July, there was a sudden upsurge: during the last week alone 133 people died.

The parish of St James, however, seemed set to retain its relative immunity. By the end of July the parish had seen only one case, albeit a fatal one, while in London as a whole the mortality rate swept on to reach forty-five out of every 10,000. The first sign that this privileged state of affairs would not continue came at the end of what was a hot, dry August. On Tuesday the 29th, a five-month-old baby girl at 40 Broad Street fell ill with what was said to be a 'summer diarrhoea'.

Broad Street, today called Broadwick Street, lay to the north of St James's Church in the part of the parish which clustered about Golden Square. It was, as its name suggests, a wide sort of thoroughfare and it provided a welcome contrast to the other high narrow streets of Soho. Its tall, four-storey, early Georgian terraces were built between 1700 and 1740, and during the eighteenth century it was considered a fashionable district. Now, however, it was thoroughly run down, and the houses, though highly rated, were transformed into overcrowded rookeries, each dwelling giving shelter to several families. As many as thirty individuals might live in a single house and one house, indeed, had fifty-four inhabitants. It was not uncommon for an entire family to live in a single room.

The sickness was in fact visited on a family living in such circumstances in the front kitchen of No. 40. For forty-eight hours the baby girl suffered an intractable diarrhoea as the mother struggled desperately to cope. Everywhere soiled napkins stood soaking in buckets of water. Then, as abruptly as it started, the diarrhoea stopped, but now the infant grew lethargic and exhausted, too weak even to make the effort to take feeds. Four days after falling ill she died.

There was no time for the anxiety and despair which the child's illness and rapid deterioration might have been expected to provoke. Three days before her death, during the night of Wednesday, 30 August 1854, cholera broke out in Soho with a fury never before or since experienced anywhere in the British Isles. In every adjacent street and alleyway people fell ill and collapsed. In Broad Street itself, fifty-six died from cholera during the last forty-eight hours of the infant's life. By 2 September the deadhouse at the workhouse, just round the corner in Poland Street, already contained eighty-two bodies.

Throughout Soho the disease struck indiscriminately at men and women, young and old, but inevitably finding a majority of victims among the tradespeople who crowded the district, from the families of tailors, shoemakers, general labourers, domestic servants, porters and messengers. Sometimes it began gradually with an insidious, mild diarrhoea that caused discomfort and inconvenience for a week or more before the true nature of the illness declared itself. More often it came precipitately, catching its victim in street or lodging-house, workshop or tavern, starting with a sudden weakness, uneasiness and perspiration, a feeling of faintness, an unsteadiness of the limbs. There might be a fluttering in the abdomen, a sense of weight or constriction about the waist, before there came 'a prodigious evacuation when the whole of the intestine seemed to be emptied at once'. Again and again fluid poured from the body, flooding through clothes and rags, soaking bedding and sheets, leaving the sufferer tossing about in an agony of abdominal cramps.

Soon there followed a desperate thirst, a craving for water often frustrated by violent bouts of vomiting and retching. Within hours the diarrhoeal motions had become an odourless white liquid that ran effortlessly from the patient – the 'rice-water stools' which were a classic diagnostic feature. A microscopic examination would have shown that these contained shreds and fragments of mucosa from the lining of the intestine.

Even now recovery was possible; the symptoms might subside and an uncertain, frightened convalescence set in. For the more badly afflicted, however, worse was to follow. As the body was sucked dry of its fluids, sudden spasms and rheumatic pains seized on the limbs. To those who watched it appeared that the sufferer was shrinking away, the body weight disappearing pound by pound, the eyes slowly receding into deep hollows, dry skin stretching into loose, inelastic folds over a shrunken abdomen. The flesh had, to the touch, already taken on the cold 'putty-like' consistency of death. If the skin was cut it sometimes failed to bleed. In the most severe cases it seemed that the victim was shrivelling away into a 'wizened monkey'. Even the complexion changed, a blueish tinge appearing which gradually deepened until it was almost black.

At length all trace of the thready uncertain pulse fell still. Now the sufferer lay in a profound, exhausted trance. At intervals eyes would be opened, a few lucid words whispered, and it seemed to onlookers that the victim was aware of everything except his own immediate danger. At last even this partial awareness slipped away to be replaced by a transient coma and ultimately by death. All too often relatives who had cared for the patient were, by this stage, themselves falling ill.

Every hospital within reach of Soho was under siege. The Middlesex Hospital admitted 120 cases of cholera in three days, 80 per cent of these coming from the parish of St James. The overwhelmed nursing staff had to be reinforced by employing temporary nurses. Among the extra staff was Florence Nightingale, a 33-year-old superintendent of a nursing home in Harley Street. Almost at once she found herself working without a break from the afternoon of Friday, 1 September, until the afternoon of Sunday the 3rd. In a letter to Mrs Gaskell she wrote: 'one poor girl, loathsomely filthy, came in and was dead in hours. I held her in my arms and I heard her saying something. I bent down to hear: "Pray God you may never be in the despair I am in at this time." ' At University College Hospital, the Charing Cross Hospital and the Workhouse Infirmary the story was the same. For most sufferers, however, hospital was out of the question. They contracted the disease, suffered and either died or recovered in their own homes. For the weary doctors hurrying from case to case, it seemed there was no specific remedy, nothing which brought relief. Whether in hospital or at home, over two thirds of cholera victims died, and died horribly.

On Saturday, 2 September, factories throughout Soho closed their doors and the population of the district began to decamp. Those who rented furnished accommodation left at once. Tenants who had furniture and possessions followed within a day or so, leaving goods to be collected once they had found fresh rooms in another part of town. Many lodging-houses were closed completely, their proprietors having died. Finally even the tradesmen sent their families away. Within a week of the start of the epidemic one eyewitness was noting how the most afflicted streets of the area were deserted by at least three quarters of their inhabitants.

By 3 September it was generally agreed among those who had seen most of the epidemic, the doctors and clergy, that there were signs of abatement. Fewer people were being attacked and the symptoms which occurred were less severe. On Friday, 8 September, the Rev. Henry Whitehead, the young curate at St Luke's Church in nearby Berwick Street, looked down on the remnants of his congregation and found it to consist mainly of poor, elderly women who lived by themselves. From his pulpit he congratulated them on their remarkable immunity. Yet even now the disease swung about and struck once again at the family in the front kitchen at No. 40. The father of the five-month-old baby girl, a police-man, caught cholera and died.

By Sunday the 10th, however, the epidemic had practically run its course. At its peak, 143 people in the parish had perished in a single day. On the 11th, only one death occurred. By 15 September the yellow 'plague' flags hung at the ends of streets to give warning of pestilence had been removed and *The Times* was publishing an eyewitness account from a reporter who ventured into the 'cholera area':

The outbreak of cholera in the vicinity of Golden Square is now subsiding but the passenger through the streets which compass that district will see many evidences of the alarming severity of the attack. Men and women in mourning are to be found in great numbers, and the chief topic of conversation is the recent epi-demic . . . An oil shop puts forth a large cask at its door, labelled in gigantic capitals 'Chloride of Lime'. The most remarkable evidence of all, however, and the most important, consists in the continual presence of lime in the roadways. The puddles are white and milky with it; great splashes of it lie about in the gutters, and the air is redolent with its strong and not very agreeable odour. The parish authorities have very wisely determined to wash all the streets of the tainted district with this powerful disinfectant; accordingly the purification takes place regularly every evening. The shop keepers have dismal stories to tell – how they would hear in the evening that one of their neighbours whom they had been talking with in the morning had expired after a few hours of agony and torture. It has even been asserted that the number of corpses was so great that they were removed wholesale in dead-carts for want of sufficient hearses to convey them; but let us hope this is incorrect.

In a little under two weeks nearly 700 people had died of cholera within the vicinity of Golden Square, and a report in the *Medical Times and Gazette* confirmed that it had indeed been necessary for the dead to be transported in carts.

Apart from its exceptional severity, two things only set the Broad Street epidemic apart from a multitude of other such outbreaks which occurred across the world during the nineteenth century. The first was the intervention of an awkward, rather diffident doctor called John Snow, the second a remarkable response from the vestry of St James's Church, Westminster.

Dr Snow lived at 18 Sackville Street, Piccadilly, in the southern part of the parish, his house barely a ten-minute walk from Broad Street. He was forty-one and a bachelor, a precise man, tidy in habit, punctilious to the point of fussiness, and seeming virtually submerged in reticence. Yet, despite his difficulties in establishing easy relationships with those about him, he had an original and interesting turn of mind. He held to his views with single-minded determination, being a lifelong teetotaller and vegetarian, relinquishing the latter practice only when his health began to fail and it occurred to him that it was inconsistent to refuse meat yet wear leather boots.

In spite of his shyness, however, John Snow had already carved out for himself a special niche in medical practice. Within weeks of the first successful anaesthetic being administered in Boston in October 1846, he established himself as a professional anaesthetist. Inventing and building his own equipment, he also devoted himself to a pioneer exploration and definition of the stages of anaesthesia. By September 1847 he was publishing an impeccable account of ether anaesthesia. Yet not until the eighth day of the cholera outbreak did the authorities in the parish of St James become aware that John Snow had a special interest in this particular disease.

The Board of Guardians met at frequent intervals throughout the crisis to organize relief. On this particular evening, Thursday, 7 September, its deliberations were interrupted by a request that Dr John Snow be admitted and allowed to address the meeting. Slightly surprised, the board nevertheless agreed and, almost before it had time to grasp what was happening, found itself being lectured by an earnest, middle-aged man who was hardly an inspiring orator. His voice has been described by his friends as husky, his words as difficult to follow, and it must therefore have been some moments before the guardians realized they were hearing some very peculiar theories about the causes of cholera.

In essence, Snow's views were remarkably simple. Cholera was undoubtedly a communicable disease, so how was it conveyed from person to person? What came from a cholera victim to make a healthy person suddenly fall ill? It seemed to John Snow that, whatever caused the disease, the commonly so-called 'cholera poison' must enter the body through mouth and intestines; in other words, it needed to be swallowed. This was based on direct observation that the intestines were the first part of the body to develop symptoms. Diarrhoea and vomiting preceded the more general effects of fever and dehydration. If 'cholera poison' was inhaled as a miasma, as popular opinion declared, the general symptoms should surely have come before the bowel disturbance.

'Cholera poison', he therefore argued, must be excreted in the profuse, colourless, watery diarrhoea that flooded from a victim. Once this almost colourless fluid dried on clothing or sheets, it became practically invisible, and hence the hands of the nurses or relatives could easily become contaminated through handling the soiled linen. Unless strict cleanliness was observed, the 'cholera poison' could then be transferred from hands to food, so reaching mouth, stomach and intestines in a fresh victim. In overcrowded circumstances, unless the strictest hygiene was observed, any patient with cholera must almost inevitably give rise to other cases within the same household. Moreover, he made the startling suggestion that the 'poison' might similarly be carried to food by flies.

The ultimate, most revolutionary step in his reasoning was, however, yet to come. The 'cholera poison', he argued, must eventually contaminate water supplies since sewers drained into the rivers which were the source of much drinking-water. He could even visualize the 'cholera poison' being washed down through the soil from leaky cesspools and sewers, so making wells polluted. While small domestic outbreaks might be explained by a direct contact with a cholera victim, the actual epidemics could only be caused by a contaminated water supply.

John Snow clearly thought of the 'cholera poison' as consisting of microscopic particles, small enough to be carried on the feet of a fly, yet potent enough for even this minute quantity to cause the disease. If his theories were correct, the 'cholera poison', if accidentally swallowed, then proliferated within the intestines of the sufferer so that large amounts were produced and excreted. He went so far as to hazard a guess as to the nature of the poison, though it was not yet identifiable under a microscope, saying that in view of its power of rapid proliferation, it must have an organized structure and could even be a cell.

John Snow's eccentric theories were not arrived at hastily. Like many doctors of his time, he had gained considerable experience of cholera, both as a nineteen-year-old medical apprentice in Newcastle upon Tyne during the 1831 epidemic and in London in 1848–9 during the second outbreak. In 1849 he set down his unorthodox opinions in a short pamphlet, *On the Mode of Communication of Cholera*. It received a polite but critical reception, for his ingenious hypothesis remained totally unproved. He could do nothing but wait for cholera to return, and was now intent on finding his proof. He was already engaged in a statistical investigation in south London to compare the incidence of cholera in households which drew drinking-water from various water companies. It was an urgent and demanding task, but he could hardly ignore the sudden explosive eruption of a cholera epidemic on his own doorstep.

Looking first at Soho's water sources, he found that the district was blessed with a superfluity of supplies. Since 1850, every house had been on the mains. Berwick Street and the eastern area were supplied by the New River Company, which brought its water from Hertfordshire, while Golden Square and the western area were serviced by the Grand Junction Water Company, drawing supplies from the Thames at Kew. Both companies turned on their mains for two hours a day, though nothing was supplied on Sundays. Each household therefore needed to collect and store its day's supply in a cistern or water-butt, either in the basement or the yard, the water pressure not being high enough to raise it above ground-floor level. Few of these butts or cisterns were regularly cleaned or supplied with a cover, and so the stores of water tended to be generally unsavoury if not positively unclean.

Yet the parish of St James had one advantage over many other overcrowded districts of London where Sunday became a day of drought, the mains supply being cut off and water needing to be begged from more far-sighted neighbours or carried a considerable distance. Underneath the parish, twenty-five to thirty feet beneath its subsoil of sand and light gravel, lay a stratum of impervious clay. Shallow surface wells therefore produced abundant water, and on street corners throughout the district there stood large cast-iron parish pumps from which a supply was always available. At least a dozen such pumps lay within a quarter-mile radius of Broad Street.

The Broad Street pump itself stood on the corner of Broad Street and Cambridge Street. It was a pump with a high reputation, for its water was invariably cool and showed a singularly clear, crystal brightness. Many considered it to supply the most palatable water available. A ladle attached to the handle meant that children and passers-by could pause and drink, and it was widely used in coffee-houses and dining-rooms, in the public houses to mix with spirits, and even by various little street-shops, where it was sold, with a teaspoonful of effervescing powder stirred in, as sherbet. The water from the Broad Street pump in fact enjoyed a metropolitan reputation.

It was therefore ironic that from the moment he became

aware of the Soho cholera outbreak, John Snow should have focused his suspicions on the water from the Broad Street pump. He visited the district and drew water from the pump. On Sunday, 3 September, the fourth day of the outbreak, it seemed so clear and bright that he felt uncertain and hesitated to act.

Nevertheless he obtained a list from the General Register Office of all deaths from cholera in the sub-districts of Golden Square, Berwick Street and St Anne's, Soho, during the week ending 2 September. Plotting these on a street map, he found a remarkable pattern of concentration. Almost all of them had occurred in a sharply defined cluster within an area no more than 500 yards in diameter. At its centre, most stricken among all the courts, alleyways and thoroughfares of Soho, lay Broad Street.

With desperate haste, Snow plunged into a belated field study. Already the factories were closed, the workmen withdrawn from the area. Even as the regular inhabitants packed their belongings and left, he began a series of door-to-door inquiries, finding himself questioning those still shaken by the sudden loss of a wife or husband, parents mourning children, employers who had seen workmen collapse in the workshop. The keeper of one coffee-shop told him she was already aware of nine of her customers being dead.

Each day he drew a sample of water from the Broad Street pump and examined it. Sometimes it was crystal clear, but at other times it seemed to contain minute white flocculent particles which proved, under the microscope, to be amorphous in form, with no definite organic structure. He noticed how if the water was allowed to stand, after a few hours it lost its 'freshness' and became flat. Gradually a film developed on its surface, and if left a couple of days it would grow positively offensive. By Thursday, 7 September, he was

convinced that the pump must be incriminated and determined to present his case to the Board of Guardians.

The parish guardians heard his views with profound
scepticism, but noted his simple proposal that the handle be
taken off the pump. With commendable open-mindedness
and despite their reservations, they saw to its removal next
morning. It needs to be emphasized that neither the Board of
Guardians nor John Snow himself ever attributed the epidemic burning itself out within the next two to three days to
this intervention. Its ferociousness was already well in
decline.

By 10 September the epidemic was over. In its aftermath
the Medical Committee of the General Board of Health
appointed three inspectors to carry out a local inquiry on
behalf of the government. The inspector paused to consider
John Snow's theories and rejected them outright. The Board
of Health report stated:

> The extraordinary eruption of cholera in the Soho district which
> was carefully examined . . . does not appear to afford any exception
> to generalizations respecting local states of uncleanliness, over-
> crowding, and imperfect ventilation. The suddenness of the out-
> break, the immediate climax and short duration, all point to some
> atmospheric or other widely diffused agent still to be discovered,
> and forbid the assumption in this instance, of any communication
> of the disease from person to person either by infection or contam-
> ination of water with the excretions of the sick.

As if to support this view, on 27 November a report came
from the Parish Paving Committee describing an investigation into the Broad Street pump, the walls of the well and its
water. The sides of the well seemed 'free of fissures or other
communications with drains or sewers by which such matters
could possibly be conveyed into the water'. Both chemical

and microscopic examination of the water had 'failed to detect anything which could be pronounced peculiar to a choleraic period or capable of acting as a predisposing, co-operating or specific agent in the production of that disease'. The Broad Street pump stood exonerated. It was flushed out by being pumped empty three times in succession and the handle was replaced.

The epidemic had died out, cholera had disappeared from the country, the Board of Health had passed judgement and the Broad Street pump was declared innocent. It therefore seems extraordinary that the committee of the St James vestry should have chosen this moment to embark on its own investigation. Reading the vestry minutes today, it is hard to detect any clear motive, but it all began on Thursday, 2 November 1854, when one of its members, Dr Edwin Lankester, had a motion accepted that 'a committee of investigation of this vestry be appointed for the purpose of investigating the causes arising out of the present sanitary conditions in the late outbreak of cholera in the districts of Golden Square and Berwick Street'. It seems probable that the thoughts of the vestry men were entirely practical and that they recognized the need for an urgent assessment of their parish's sanitary conditions and for a series of recommendations to improve them.

On the 23rd of the month, after some discussion, Dr Lankester's vaguely defined motion was formally approved, and nine vestry men, including Dr Lankester and the church wardens, were appointed committee members. Almost at once there was consternation in the parish. On 16 December, the vestry was obliged to debate the matter yet again after a letter from the Board of Guardians complained not only of the expense of such an inquiry, but also *of the mischievous effects which a renewed investigation of the subject so recently made by the Government's Officers is calculated to inflict on the Householders and Inhabitants of the locality, now but slowly recovering from the serious depression of their trade and employment and by whom the inquiry instituted by the vestry is consequently viewed with feelings of dissatisfaction and alarm.*

It took some considerable argument before the proposal to disband the committee was rejected.

Having weathered these early storms, the committee got down to attempting to review all information already collected. This proved unexpectedly difficult. Sir Benjamin Hall, chairman of the Board of Health, whose government inspectors had already visited the parish, met its request bluntly and dismissively. He declined to make available any information gathered by his department on the grounds that 'investigations of this kind were more valuable when independent'.

Nonplussed but undeterred, the committee obstinately set about gathering its own information. A questionnaire asking about detailed living circumstances was drawn up, printed and distributed to every household in the district. A vast majority of these circulars was never seen again. 'This measure did not produce the anticipated results,' the committee gravely noted. There was no alternative to a comprehensive series of personal interviews with householders. But such an ambitious undertaking demanded more help, and it was decided to co-opt eight further members. The committee therefore almost doubled in size, and now included, besides numerous vestry men, six doctors and two clergymen. Among the new members were the Rev. Henry Whitehead, curate of St Luke's, and Dr John Snow.

John Snow had not been idle. In the bare three months since the cholera outbreak he had expanded his original thirty-page pamphlet on cholera into a 162-page book. It now contained not only an account of his researches in south London but also a graphic description of the Soho outbreak. So far as John Snow was concerned, his hypothesis was beyond dispute. It must have been somewhat galling to find that scarcely any other committee member believed a word of it. He went so far as to present a copy to the Rev. Whitehead, and received in return a letter of thanks politely pointing out the reasons why the curate thought the hypothesis untenable.

Nevertheless the committee prepared to forge ahead. Each member was to conduct a door-to-door inquiry in one particular street, John Snow being allocated the rather small and relatively lightly afflicted Peter Street. Henry Whitehead, by now energetically determined to disprove Snow's hypothesis, had volunteered for the awesome task of investigating Broad Street, itself known to have close on a thousand inhabitants.

One of the most striking features of the Soho epidemic was its sharply limited extent, both in time and geographical spread. Over several weeks there had been an occasional case of cholera in the district until quite suddenly, during the night of Monday, 30 August, there was virtually an explosion of cholera with few streets or houses escaping. A fortnight later it was practically over. Similarly, in the midst of the intricate tangle of back streets, alleyways and courtyards, it was possible to say that the 'cholera area' stopped half-way along a given street or that it included only one side of a certain square. Almost more intriguing were the so-called 'eccentricities' of the disease. Within the 'cholera area', one house in the middle of a row might stand entirely untouched. The workhouse in Poland Street, for instance, where the bodies of cholera victims were brought each day to the deadhouse and scores of dying patients were admitted to the infirmary, escaped practically unscathed. Only five of its 535 regular inmates died during the epidemic.

The Committee of Inquiry remained convinced that there had to be a local factor to account for the pattern of this peculiarly intense, restricted outbreak. How, on the night of 30 August 1854, had Broad Street and its neighbouring thoroughfares provided such dry tinder for the spark of cholera? In what way had the area's streets, houses or even inhabitants differed from those in crowded districts which escaped comparatively unscathed on every side?

The elevation of various streets; the nature of the soil and subsoil; the surface and ground plan of the district; the arrangements of the houses and courts; the density and character of the population; even the internal economy of the individual houses – none of these things was left out of account. The site and conditions of sewers, the effectiveness of house drains, the continued survival of old cesspools – all were examined. The Rev. Henry Whitehead, with naïve distaste, had been under the impression that most cesspools were abolished. His door-to-door inquiries soon showed, however, that most houses still had privies, usually in the basement yard, sometimes in the front area but only occasionally within the house itself. Water closets were rare. Most privies had a bar rather than a seat, and they nearly all stank for they stood, without any form of water-trap, directly over cesspools that were rarely emptied.

Smaller children found the bars in the privies too high and tended to use the open yards. In attic rooms the inconvenience of reaching a privy four storeys below encouraged some tenants to empty slops on to the roofs so that miniature cesspools formed in guttering. The cesspools which drained the privies were supposed to have been filled in when new

sewers were laid, but since they still existed, it was the actual
overflow from them which spilled into the sewers, and these
were hardly less offensive.

Of the district's three main sewage systems, one was very
old, but the others had been laid quite recently, the last only
a few months before the epidemic. All of them featured open
ventilating grills, untrapped gullies and an exceedingly gentle
gradient with a fall of only 1 in 250. Their untreated contents
were discharged straight into the Thames at the end of
Northumberland Avenue, close to Charing Cross, and at high
tide it was common for sewage to come flooding back into
the drains.

The generally held theory that cholera was transmitted by
'effluvia' would seem to have been supported by the fact that
Soho abounded in unpleasant odours. Smells emanated from
the sewers, from rotting garbage and refuse, from overcrowded, filthy houses, and from a variety of pungent trades
and industries. Apart from a wholesale abattoir, where blood
was allowed to run down to the gutters and animals' intestines were left outside for collection, at least eight butchers
kept and slaughtered their own cattle. There was also a bone-
boiling factory, a brewery and a tripe house. The stifling
summer weather, the narrow thoroughfares and the tall
houses which hindered the circulation of fresh air must have
made conditions almost intolerable. As the Committee of
Inquiry observed, however, this was 'a fault common to most
parts of London and other towns'. There was 'nothing
peculiar in the sewers or drainage of the limited spot in
which the outbreak occurred; and Saffron Hill and other
locations which suffer much more from ill odours, have been
very lightly visited by the cholera'.

Not even the simple equation of dirt with disease stood up
to scrutiny. Three houses congratulated by the parochial

authorities for their outstanding cleanliness were almost the only ones in a certain street to be visited by the disease, one of them losing twelve inhabitants. In ironic contrast, the most appallingly dirt-ridden house in the neighbourhood was alone in a terrace of forty-five to escape without a death. 'Want of cleanliness', said Henry Whitehead drily, 'was by no means more characteristic of the diseased than of the survivors.'

Florence Nightingale had remarked: 'The prostitutes came in perpetually, poor creatures staggering off their beat: it took worse hold of them than any.' Yet Henry Whitehead, having spent several months investigating, was unable to reach such a clear-cut conclusion: 'Again there is no ground for saying in this epidemic that the intemperate suffered worse than the temperate, the poor than the rich, the weak than the strong. In short those best acquainted with the district were altogether unable to trace any connexion between the disease and the habits and circumstances of the people it attacked.'

Moreover, he wrote, no satisfactory explanation had emerged to account for the 'sharp line of demarcation' which surrounded the 'cholera area', while the 'apparent anomalies within the area itself' remained beyond explanation. The Committee of Inquiry was at an impasse.

Mr Whitehead, having set out specifically to disprove John Snow's theory, had laboured mightily in Broad Street. His survey of the street's inhabitants was, for its time, one of the most intensive and meticulous pieces of research ever undertaken. He had been determined to interview every family resident at the moment of outbreak. Where families moved away, he attempted to contact them, in some cases travelling considerable distances. With those that remained he went over the ground again and again, sometimes visiting a family four or five times. He managed to speak to 497 of the 896 original inhabitants, collecting detailed information about not only the ninety residents and the twenty-eight non-resident factory workers who had died, but also about those who had suffered from the disease and recovered. Thus he gathered accurate records for every case of cholera in Broad Street, the names and ages of victims, situations of rooms occupied, sanitary arrangements, water drunk and the exact hour of onset.

And as the information accumulated, so Whitehead was forced to recognize that Snow was right: the Broad Street pump was somehow directly implicated. Of 137 persons in Broad Street who drank water from the pump, eighty developed cholera. Among 297 who did not use the pump, only twenty suffered. For the first time Whitehead understood the immunity of the solitary old women of his congregation: they had no one to send to the pump for water.

John Snow had pointed out that the Broad Street pump stood at the heart of the 'cholera area', with the epidemic extending outward only as far as that point where it became easier to fetch water from another pump. In the occasional houses contaminated by cholera beyond that boundary, it was possible to show that their inhabitants had made a point of fetching water from Broad Street. If the workhouse in Poland Street in the centre of the 'cholera area' had escaped, it now seemed that no thanks were owing to its enforced hygiene and spartan wards. It had its own pump upon the premises, as well as a mains supply from the Grand Junction Company, and did not need to use the Broad Street pump. Similarly, at the brewery in Broad Street, not one of the seventy brewer's men had suffered. Mr Huggins, the proprietor, was positive that none of his employees used the Broad Street pump. The brewery, he told John Snow, had its own deep well and received a mains supply from the New River

Water Company, besides which each workman was entitled to an allowance of malt liquor.

At the Eley Percussion Cap Factory at No. 37, however, eighteen had died out of the workforce of 200, and here two large tubs of drinking-water were kept replenished from the street pump. There was also the curious case of Mrs Susannah Eley, widow of the founder. She had retired to Hampstead but still preferred the water from Broad Street. Her sons, who ran the company, would therefore send her a large bottle of it each day by carrier's cart. On 1 September Mrs Eley was seized with cholera; the next day she died. A visiting niece from Islington also died, but no other cases of cholera came to light in Hampstead or Islington.

John Snow in fact discovered a succession of instances parallel to that of Mrs Eley, and his original condemnation of the Broad Street pump stood vindicated. Thus far the medical authorities were prepared to travel with him. The effluvium of cholera was thought to be fermented from decaying matter or stagnant water and it was in any case already accepted in the Registrar-General's returns that a high incidence of cholera mortality was often associated with an impure water supply. Without exception, however, the most distinguished experts still thought the idea preposterous that leaks of faecal matter could be responsible. The Scientific Committee of the General Board of Health, when it reported in 1854, reaffirmed its acceptance of 'the doctrine that the exciting cause of cholera is something which acts in the manner of a ferment, that it, therefore, takes effect only amid congenial circumstances and that the stuff out of which it bears poison must be air or water abounding with organic impurity'.

Dr Hassall, who had carried out the microscopic examination of water samples for the Scientific Committee, was openly scornful of the popular idea that 'everything we eat or drink teems with life, and that even our bodies abound with minute living and parasitic productions. This is a vulgar error and the notion is as disgusting as it is erroneous.' The Scientific Committee itself would concede nothing concerning 'Dr Snow's suggestion that the real cause lay in the use of a particular well, whose waters were contaminated with rice water evacuation of cholera patients'. It came to accept that the well-water did 'really act as the vehicle of choleraic infection', but saw no reason to agree that 'infection depended on the specific material alleged'. The Royal College of Physicians stood firmly behind this conclusion.

In St James, the parish Paving Committee had, of course, already stated that it could find no way in which such contamination might have occurred. And the fact remained that John Snow had been able to produce no shred of evidence, beyond assumptions, to show how the well-water became dangerous. Nevertheless, St James's Committee of Inquiry continued to discuss the possibility of sewage having somehow percolated into the well, even though it had no proof. Not until 3 April 1855 did the Rev. Henry Whitehead stumble over the missing piece of the jigsaw. A brief entry in the Registrar-General's return of deaths suddenly caught his attention with a glaring significance:

At 40 Broad Street, 2nd September, a daughter, aged five months, exhaustion after an attack of diarrhoea four days previous to death.

No. 40 was the house adjacent to the Broad Street pump, and here was a case of severe diarrhoea which commenced forty-eight hours before the Soho outbreak. Whitehead hurried round to the address and heard how the mother had steeped her baby's soiled napkins in pails of water, emptying these into the privy at the front of the house. This privy stood only a few feet away from the pump, and Whitehead lost no time in placing his discovery before the committee. An immediate re-examination of the cesspool and well was ordered, and the findings were horrific.

The main drain, when opened for inspection, proved to be an old-fashioned, flat-bottomed gully a foot wide and a foot deep, covered by stone slabs. Two inches of sludge lay in its bottom as its gradient was incorrectly linked to the sewer and so was inadequate. The bricks and mortar in its walls had decayed so that individual bricks could be lifted freely from their bedding. Hence the drain leaked like a sieve.

Further back towards the house, connecting with the drain and built of the same decayed brickwork, a cesspool was discovered which served the open privy. This cesspool, supposed to act as a trap, was also wrongly constructed and had become so full that it not only leaked through its porous brickwork but overflowed and saturated the wooden boards which covered it. The cesspool had clearly been in this condition for many months.

The sides of the drain were found to pass less than three feet from the sides of the well. The bottom of the drain stood nine feet above the well's normal water level. The brickwork of the well's wall was laid in the usual manner, without mortar, so that water could percolate through the bricks from the surrounding gravel subsoil. Sample probings into the walls showed that this gravel was rich in human slurry.

Whitehead and the Committee of Inquiry now felt certain that the baby girl who fell ill in the front kitchen of 40 Broad Street was the primary cause of the outbreak. Even so, Whitehead was still puzzled by the way the cholera subsided so quickly. There had been other cases at No. 40: two men and a woman. How did their rice-water stools evade soaking down to the well and sustaining the epidemic? These patients had been nursed in an upstairs room at the back of the house, and under cross-questioning their relatives confessed to Mr Whitehead that it had been easier to fling slops from the back window than carry them downstairs to the privy.

Finally Whitehead noticed how, on 8 September, the father of the infant girl contracted cholera and died within twenty-four hours. Nursed in the front kitchen, he had used the front privy. His excretions must have contaminated the well – but it was on the day he fell ill that the pump handle was removed. Thus it was realized in retrospect how John Snow directly prevented the Soho cholera epidemic from breaking out with redoubled violence.

Three months after Whitehead's discoveries, on 9 August 1855, the Cholera Inquiry Committee presented its report to the vestry. The text ran to 175 pages, contained statements by John Snow and Henry Whitehead and was presented by Dr Edwin Lankester, who, according to the vestry minutes, 'brought up a report thereof at considerable length and read a portion as well as stated the general character and contents of the same'. The report was carefully drafted, the evidence impartially presented and the conclusions cautious and strictly defined:

Anxious to give due weight to every fact and consideration that have offered themselves in the inquiry, the Committee is unanimously of the conclusion that the striking disproportionate mortality in the 'cholera area' as compared with the immediately surrounding districts, which constitutes the sudden, severe and concentrated outbreaks, beginning on August 31st, and lasting for a few early days of September, was in some measure attributable to the use of the impure water of the well in Broad Street.

While the committee refrained from expressing an opinion in favour of any one hypothesis, its recommendations were simple but quite revolutionary: all surface wells should be abolished, all cisterns should be removed and the water companies should provide a continuous supply of water. Furthermore, stand-pipes connected to the mains should be erected in the streets to provide free water.

It was not at all what the vestry had expected. The report and its recommendations provoked a heated debate, and, when the question of acceptance arose, the votes for and against were exactly equal. The stalemate was resolved by the vestry chairman, Mr William Geesin, who used his casting vote in favour of the report. Despite protests from the Board of Guardians about the expense, it was decided to print 200 copies for general sale. The publication was a commercial failure. Nine months later, the vestry needed to request £170 12s. 7d. from the poor rate to cover the inquiry's costs.

Despite the Committee of Inquiry's unequivocal recommendations, it was several years before any of them were put into effect. Indeed, not until 1866, after repeated protests from Dr Lankester, then medical officer to the parish, and with the threat of yet another epidemic imminent, was the Broad Street pump itself finally abolished.

John Snow sold no more than fifty-six copies of his book *On the Mode of Communication of Cholera*. It had cost him more than £200 to prepare and publish, but earned him only £3 12s. Sadly, he never lived to see his work on cholera acclaimed. On 16 June 1858, aged forty-four, he was overwhelmed by a fatal stroke within minutes of writing the closing lines of his third great book, a treatise on the use of chloroform as an anaesthetic.

After his death his theories on cholera came to be re-examined with increasing respect. As one medical authority, J. Netten Radcliffe, wrote in 1871, Snow's doctrine of the transmission of cholera through polluted water was 'now fully accepted in medicine'. But, he added, 'to Mr Whitehead unquestionably belongs the honour of having first shown . . . the high degree of probability attaching to it. Only now perhaps can the great public importance of the doctrine be clearly appreciated, and the value of Mr Whitehead's inquiry properly estimated.'

Henry Whitehead was in the forefront of the next battle against cholera when the disease returned to London in 1866. It is said that the Editor of the *Daily News* asked: 'Is there not a small bishopric for such a man?' It was not to be. Having served as curate and vicar in several London parishes, Whitehead accepted a living at Bramford, a small town in Cumberland. He died at Lanercost Priory on 5 March 1896 at the age of seventy.

In 1884, the keystone in the edifice of Snow's hypothesis fell into place when the great German bacteriologist Robert Koch identified the germ responsible, the cholera vibrio. This organism, in mode of action and transmission, fulfilled every detail of the theoretical picture of a 'cholera poison' which John Snow had built up more than thirty years before. The discovery was in effect the fulfilment of a prophecy.

Today the Committee of Inquiry appointed by St James's vestry is virtually forgotten while the name of the Rev. Henry Whitehead rests in decent obscurity. Only on John Snow has a posthumous honour been bestowed. In Soho, on a corner in Broadwick Street, formerly Broad Street, the John Snow Tavern occupies the site overlooking the spot where the Broad Street pump once stood, for, to the dismay of his family, his fellow countrymen have with a perverse but sincere respect celebrated that dedicated teetotaller by giving his name to a public house.

Chapter 6

A Fallen Splendour

The American Embassy in Rome is housed in the Palazzo Margherita, which stands where the Via Veneto turns down into the lower city. When Italy was still a monarchy, this elegant palace had been the residence of the Queen Mother: a place of courtyards and marble stairways, of grand rooms leading off long corridors. The ambassador's office on the second floor was once the Queen Mother's dining room, its décor of white and gold set off by a chandelier of Venetian glass. The ambassador's desk is placed before tall windows which look down on to the heat, dust and traffic of the Via Veneto, while to the right of the ambassador's chair stands the flag of the United States of America, and, to the left, the personal ambassadorial flag of forty-eight stars set on a field of blue.

The official residence of the ambassador is not here, however, but a quarter of an hour's drive away at the Villa Taverna, a secluded late-seventeenth-century palace in the north of the city. Tucked away behind high stone walls and approached through a long tunnel of intertwining olive boughs, it stands in a seven-acre garden of close-cropped lawns, formal flower beds, fountains, marble statues, and tall ilex and cypress trees. It was built in 1690 for a cardinal, then used, for a time, as a Jesuit seminary before becoming the abode of a succession of counts and princes. Ultimately, in

1948, the US Government bought it for the use of its ambassador.

It is now February 1953, and the new US President, Dwight D. Eisenhower, has broken with tradition and nominated a small, deceptively fragile-looking woman, with golden hair, blue eyes and attractive features, to be America's ambassador in Rome. It is a controversial appointment. Mrs Clare Boothe Luce is a notable convert to Catholicism, and in the United States there is widespread concern among Protestant organizations that she could be unduly influenced by the Vatican. Furthermore, although the American tide of anti-Communist feeling is running high, with Senator Joseph McCarthy steering his Sub-committee for Un-American Activities towards its climax, in Italy Communism is an established political force. The Partido Comunista Italiano is the largest national Communist party outside the Communist states, and there is among Italians consternation that the new ambassador should be a congresswoman known for her outspokenness against Communism. Neither does the fact of her being a woman help; only seven years have gone by since Italian women gained the franchise.

Despite the difficulties of the assignment, the appointment is for Mrs Luce the crown to a successful and varied career. As a journalist, she rose to become managing editor of the magazine *Vanity Fair*. As an author, she has written filmscripts as well as several Broadway hits. As a war-correspondent, she has travelled throughout Europe and Asia, interviewing and becoming acquainted with most of the leading figures of her day. And as a congresswoman, she has served twice for the 4th Congressional District of Connecticut. Her first, early marriage may have been a failure, but she has subsequently made up for that by marrying Henry Luce, proprietor, publisher and editor of *Life* magazine. She is a hard-hitting public speaker who projects her views with pugnacious wit and candour, and a Gallup Poll has just declared her to be the fourth most admired woman in the world after Eleanor Roosevelt, Queen Elizabeth II and Mrs Dwight D. Eisenhower.

On 17 February, she testifies before a closed hearing of the Senate Foreign Relations Committee that she supports 'the American tradition of separation of Church and State' and that in her new post she will 'have no relations, formal or informal, open or secret' with the Vatican. On 2 March, the Senate confirms her appointment. On 16 April, six days after her fiftieth birthday, she arrives in Rome to face her greatest challenge.

When Mrs Luce arrived to take up residence at the Villa Taverna, she found a certain austerity about its great vaulted entrance hall and formal rooms – 'As cosy as a half-filled mausoleum' was how one writer described it – and at once felt the need to send home for her own paintings, carpets and furnishings. Her private quarters, on the second floor, consisted of a study and a large adjoining bedroom. With the spaciousness of the study she fell in love, especially with its high, heavy-beamed ceiling, the dark green of which was relieved by cluster upon cluster of resplendent white stucco roses and rosettes. This ceiling had been much admired by her predecessors as a fine example of Italian Renaissance decoration. Aware of the long hours and mountains of paperwork awaiting her, she decided therefore to convert the study into a study-bedroom, surrendering the quiet privacy of the bedroom to her husband, come to see her safely installed but battling to maintain herculean work schedules 2,000 miles from his publishing empire.

The situation which confronted Clare Boothe Luce was

appallingly complex. Italian politics were in a phase of exceptional instability. Twenty-one years of Fascist dictatorship had ended with the country defeated and reduced to a battleground for contending foreign armies, with the Vatican, throughout the turmoil, seeking to maintain an uneasy neutrality. Barely eight years had passed since the country had regained control of its own destiny, and now to be left wing was to be Communist, to be right wing was to be accused of being Fascist, and to be moderate was to pick a wavering path between fine shades of political opinion. To be American was to be both conqueror and liberator, benevolent and paternalistic, authoritative and interfering, selfrighteous and self-assured, and, above all, stridently anti-Communist. It was not an easy role to fill with grace in a country of volatile temperaments, religious enthusiasm and bitter memories. America, it seemed, was trying to teach politics and diplomacy to the land that produced Machiavelli.

The monarchist newspaper *Candido* celebrated the new ambassador's arrival with a cartoon of the US Embassy flying a stars and stripes edged with lace. Yet while she needed, on the one hand, to overcome the prejudices and hostility of Italian diplomatic circles, she faced, on the other, the half-hidden resentments of her own staff, for, almost worse than being a woman, she was a Republican. With the Republicans having been returned to power after twenty years of Democratic victories in the United States, the 300 individuals who staffed the embassy and the 1,000 or so employed in official US legations, organizations and agencies throughout the country, could only see the new ambassador, representing the new administration, as a portent of change. There was uncertainty over jobs and anxiety about future careers. Within days of her arrival the official press attaché had indeed been replaced.

At the start of her ambassadorship, she threw an impromptu garden party at the Villa Taverna for all those who worked in the embassy, many of whom had never seen the official residence. That done with, she buried herself in an unbroken round of work. From the moment she opened her eyes each morning and stared up at the cluster upon cluster of white stucco roses, entwining across the dark-green beams of the study ceiling, to the moment of sinking back exhausted into the cool softness of her bed, she was on duty. She was roused each day at 7 a.m. by the noise and vibration of the heavy washing-machine in the third-floor laundry room immediately overhead. At eight the breakfast tray arrived as she lay in bed, reading the mail, dictating replies into a machine or learning Italian from tape-recorded lessons. Sipping a second cup of coffee, she would ponder on her carefully timed schedule, and at 9.45 precisely leave for the embassy in a chauffeur-driven blue Cadillac. By ten o'clock she would be beginning the first of her engagements, returning to the Villa Taverna at 1.30 for lunch and a brief but incisive planning discussion with the staff. At 3 p.m. the succession of interviews and appointments began again, and at 7 p.m. she returned home, usually to change for a fleeting courtesy visit to some diplomatic cocktail party before changing yet again to grace a formal dinner which might well continue till midnight with a succession of speeches to be endured and a careful ritual of diplomatic protocol to be observed. Finally, alone in her room at last, she would allow herself to unwind, studying the last of the urgent dispatches brought up from the embassy or quietly writing her diary. She was rarely in bed before one or two in the morning.

As American ambassador to Italy she had set herself three objectives. The first was, quite simply, to foster good relations between the two countries. The second was to help with finding a solution to the apparently insoluble problem of the future of the city of Trieste. The third was, in her own forthright words, 'to aid by every proper means the young democratic republic of Italy to fight the malignant growth of Communism in the Italian body politic'.

It was on 5 May, less than three weeks after her arrival, that Clare Boothe Luce made her first major speech in Italy, and with it her first mistake. As guest of honour at a dinner given by the Milanese Chamber of Commerce, she spoke of her host-country with enthusiasm and admiration: 'In Italy's thrilling forward progress along the ancient highway of her natural greatness, she can count confidently on America's intimate and warm co-operation.' Yet in the midst of the high-flown phrases there crouched the blunder. 'But if . . . the Italian people should fall the unhappy victims of totalitarianism, totalitarianism of the right or of the left, there would follow, logically and tragically, grave consequences for this intimate and warm co-operation we now enjoy.' The Milanese Chamber of Commerce applauded; the Italian press sounded its protests.

Communist as well as neo-Fascist newspapers throughout the country interpreted the remark as an attempt not only by Mrs Luce but also by the US Government to meddle in Italian domestic politics. Even Italians of moderate persuasion showed their resentment. The scarcely veiled suggestion of coercion provoked inevitable reaction, and in the elections which followed a few weeks later the Christian Democrats were defeated by a narrow margin, being 55,000 votes short of an absolute majority. More disturbingly for American interests, the Communist Party won 36 per cent of the vote. Government by coalition was now the only option and the Christian Democrats needed to seek an alliance with one of the other eighty-one registered political parties. Unfortunately, the first attempt at a coalition government collapsed within a fortnight.

America looked on with consternation. Perhaps Mrs Luce's speech had tipped the scales: the American ambassador spoke, the election was lost, the Communists prospered. It was rumoured she would be recalled. In Italy, there was an open hostility to the United States and its ambassador. Successive further attempts to form an administration were tried and failed. The warmth of June matured into the July heat and the unrelenting furnace of August, yet Clare Boothe Luce still found herself unable to carry on official business, there being no government with whom to negotiate.

In July, when Henry Luce returned to Rome, he was startled by his wife's appearance. She had lost weight and seemed tired; she complained of suffering from 'Roman tummy', a transient disturbance of the digestive system that had plagued generations of visitors to the city. The stomach pains and abdominal cramps, the noisy internal rumblings and sudden upheavals in her bowels, she attributed to an unaccustomed richness of food. The banquets she attended, with their succession of highly spiced dishes cooked in olive oil, had become unpleasant ordeals on account of her loss of appetite and occasional bouts of nausea. Her illness, which she regarded as nothing more serious than a regional variant on the travellers' ubiquitous gippy tummy, should have lasted hardly more than a week. Unfortunately, it had been going on for three months.

To relieve some of the pressures on her, her husband stole her away for a secluded holiday, chartering a private yacht to cruise in the Tyrrhenian Sea. Yet even here the holiday was punctuated by a steady flow of diplomatic mail. Events were not prepared to wait on the American ambassador. At last, on 15 August, a coalition, a caretaker administration, was successfully formed under the leadership of Giuseppe Pella. Thirteen days later, as the Luces' yacht lay idling in the picturesque harbour of Portofino, a message from the embassy brought their vacation abruptly to an end. The Trieste crisis had broken.

The city of Trieste occupied, with its great port, a key position at the north-east head of the Adriatic, directly on the border between Italy and Yugoslavia. Its population included a complex intermixing of peoples of Slav descent, but was predominantly Italian. Before the Second World War, Trieste had belonged to Italy, who had built up major industries there, and founded the university. In 1943, however, the city was annexed by the German Third Reich, and it came about that it was Marshall Tito's Yugoslav troops who were first among the liberating armies to enter and claim the territory in 1945.

Trieste had not been returned to Italy. Faced with the rival claims of victorious Yugoslavia and defeated Italy, the Allied Powers had sought a compromise and created the 'Free Territory of Trieste', a miniature state administered in one zone by the United States and Britain and in the other by Yugoslavia. Inevitably, the compromise failed to work, and the competing claims of Italy and Yugoslavia rumbled on as a highly sensitive issue in each country.

With the fall of the Christian Democrats in 1953 and the sequence of failed coalitions in Italy, President Tito saw his chance to make his claims more pressing. On 28 August, with the Luces still at sea, the Yugoslav News Agency issued a statement that the Yugoslav Government had lost patience with Italy's 'unconstructive behaviour' and was re-examining its attitude to the Trieste question. With considerable foreboding, the Italian Government interpreted the statement as indicating that Yugoslavia intended to annexe the whole of

Trieste. The next day Italian troops moved up to the border where Yugoslav troops were already taking up positions, and on the 30th the cruiser *Duca degli Abrizzi* with two Italian destroyers arrived at Venice from the lower Adriatic. Within a fortnight of coming to office, the new Italian coalition had reached the brink of war.

Mrs Luce plunged herself into a series of urgent meetings and consultations and a deluge of coded cables as she sought to mediate between the Eisenhower administration and the Italian Government. To the Italian leaders, she preached restraint; to the Allies, she pleaded the Italian cause. Eventually, on 8 October, the United States and Britain jointly declared that they intended to withdraw from the part of Trieste they controlled and let the Italians take over.

Marshall Tito objected at once. A crop of Italian flags instantly sprang up on buildings throughout the city and Allied commanders found themselves coping with street riots by demonstrators who wanted to see the Allies withdraw so Italian troops could take control. The rioting and looting and the destruction of vehicles and property which followed were aggravated by extremist *agents provocateurs* from Italy. Allied troops were attacked by enraged mobs, shots were exchanged. There were, inevitably, a few civilian deaths. A wave of shocked protest swept Italy.

The sixth of November saw demonstrations in Rome, Milan, Venice, Naples, Reggio Calabria and Palermo. Cars with US or British number plates were attacked and damaged; one was burned. British airline officers were assaulted in the street. On the 7th, about 12,000 youths, led by neo-Fascist deputies, marched on the United States Embassy in Rome and Mrs Luce found herself besieged by an infuriated Roman mob.

It looked as though her diplomatic career had reached its

nadir. In the few months since she had become ambassador, the elections had been lost, her name and that of her country had been subjected to execration, her embassy had come under attack. The Italian Government was permanently wracked by internal schism. The Trieste crisis was dead-locked, the Italians having announced they would not nego-tiate until they were in occupation of the city of Trieste, even as Yugoslavia stood by its ultimatum of war should Italy take over.

Mrs Luce was tired and despondent, and still suffering from her oddly persistent 'Roman tummy', yet she got off a spirited dispatch to Washington, pointing out that the popu-larity of the Communists had gone on increasing since they had polled 36 per cent of the vote in June. They needed only 4 per cent more of the vote before the Italian President would be constitutionally required to call on a Communist leader, such as Palmiro Togliatti, to form the next government. She insisted that only by resolving the Trieste crisis could America hope to stem the swing to Communism.

In December, the current Prime Minister, Giuseppe Pella, approached her discreetly to inquire whether, since the Italians refused to negotiate, the Allies might be persuaded to open secret talks with Yugoslavia to discover on what grounds Tito would allow the Italians to move into Trieste. It was the first sign of a way out, but then, within weeks, Signor Pella's coalition went the way of its predecessors. Ignoring the fate of the government, Clare Boothe Luce herself flew to Washington to lay the proposal before President Eisenhower, adding that, in her view, if they were to stand any chance of succeeding, such negotiations should be conducted not in the overheated atmosphere of Rome or Belgrade but in some neutral yet friendly capital.

By 2 February 1954, when secret negotiations began in

London between the Allies and Yugoslavia, Clare Boothe Luce was back in Rome, settled once more to the relentless round of careful decisions and formal engagements. Now she was more than ever aware of the need for an imperturbable façade, allowing no hint to escape of the tensions associated with the secret talks.

The political situation in Italy remained confused. A fresh government, formed on 18 January, had survived only twelve days. On 10 February, yet another coalition was brought together, and Mrs Luce, negotiating with the fifth Italian government of her ambassadorship, found herself almost at once under fresh attack. In a speech to the Italian Chamber of Deputies, the Communist leader, Palmiro Togliatti, accused the United States of having, through the actions of its ambassador, prevented the formation of a stable government on the basis of an understanding between Communists and Christian Democrats.

The Italian magazine *L'Europeo*, moreover, reported a speech criticizing the Italian Government which Mrs Luce supposedly made in Washington. A group of Communist and Socialist senators demanded that Mrs Luce be declared *persona non grata* and that the American Government be asked to recall her for 'interference in Italian politics and remarks offensive to the highest authorities in the state'. She could only retort that the magazine article was a 'fabrication, pure and simple'.

By 30 May, a tentative agreement was reached in London with the Yugoslav representatives. A possible basis for settlement had been defined. It was time to negotiate with spokesmen from the Italian Foreign Ministry, but by now Clare Boothe Luce was suffering from what she described as a 'bone-gnawing fatigue'. She felt the need for more sleep and contrived to spend longer in bed, yet found she only awoke feeling worse. She was conscious of an unaccustomed nervousness, a slight but definite unease. Nausea, loss of appetite and occasional stomach pains persisted. Since her breakfast coffee tasted bitter and metallic, she changed to an American brand and installed an automatic coffee-maker, complaining that Italians could not make coffee. Just as she needed her health and strength, it seemed she was being plagued by a host of ill-defined annoyances. In early June, she attended the Venice Art Festival. When a friend asked her to waltz, she found her right foot had grown inexplicably numb. She almost had to drag it as she danced.

At the end of June she started a long vacation and returned to the United States for two months, quietly entering a New York hospital for an intensive medical check-up. To her surprise, a diagnosis was made of serious anaemia and extreme nervous fatigue. To her grateful relief, the symptoms began to recede and each day found her more comfortable, her strength returning. By August, she was eager to get back into the fray. Quitting was not the style of the woman who had once accepted defeat in a congressional election campaign by stepping to the microphone and quoting Dryden:

> I will lay me down and bleed awhile,
> Then I'll rise and fight with you again.

The negotiations in London had already obtained a qualified agreement from the Italians. Now the diplomats were talking with each side simultaneously without allowing the factions to meet. But in mid-August reports came from London that negotiations had broken down.

In Rome, seated again at her desk, gazing down through the tall windows of her office on to the sun-baked oven of the Via Veneto, Clare Boothe Luce felt the tension all about her. There was a fearful expectancy in the air. The tiredness and fatigue were back, along with the familiar nervousness. And now there was a new symptom: a sense of tightness and irritability that left her at odds with everyday events. At the Villa Taverna she complained about the heaviness of the footsteps in the service quarters overhead. She listened impatiently to the polite and interesting explanation: that since the villa had been built at a time when there was a considerable fear of earthquakes, the walls were hollow so that beams and floors could be suspended on concealed chains to give flexibility and strength.

On 5 October, Clare Boothe Luce was asked to give out an official statement being issued simultaneously in Belgrade, London and Washington. The unbelievable had occurred. An agreement acceptable to the Italian and Yugoslav governments had been reached on the future of the Free Territory of Trieste. Yugoslavia was to take the whole southern zone with a small immediately adjacent strip of the northern zone. Italy was to take the remainder of the northern zone, together with the city itself and the harbour. The Trieste dispute was settled.

Italy broke out into immediate waves of rejoicing. The following day was declared an official school holiday. Newspapers showered praise on the settlement, on negotiations and negotiators, on the United States and even on the US Ambassador. The embassy was inundated with telegrams and messages of congratulation, and when Mrs Luce drove in her blue Cadillac with 'Stars and Stripes' pennant fluttering, she found passers-by waving and even calling greetings. The head of the Italian Foreign Office gave an official luncheon for those Americans in Rome who had assisted in any way with the negotiations and Mrs Luce received an unexpected presentation: her own gold cigarette-case which she thought mislaid. It had been borrowed and skilfully modified. Inlaid on its surface in brilliants and rubies was the coat of arms of the city of Trieste. The American Ambassador disgraced herself by crying.

The Trieste resolution brought a welcome and unfamiliar relaxation, but this did not seem to mitigate Mrs Luce's 'extreme nervous fatigue'. More disconcertingly, there were changes in her behaviour, several observers describing her manner as strange and claiming that, on occasions, she seemed drunk or on drugs. Wilfred Sheed, in his biography of her, quotes a letter from the writer Isabella Taves describing Mrs Luce arriving for a party in Rome:

'Madame arrives spaced out . . . it wasn't liquor, but she was being very odd. First, she went on about seeing a flying saucer on the Via Veneto, then she began on insulation of airports, at which point the other guests were palpably going nuts, so Miss Taves tried to interject a question. Clare just kept on going, this time about the future of insulated housing, winding up: "Think what it will mean to us housewives!" '

By next day she was as rational as ever.

She was also experiencing physical symptoms. Her finger nails had grown brittle and would break at a tap. When she brushed her hair, the brush became clogged with long strands of blonde hair. Her mouth and gums felt uncomfortable and she had an impression of her teeth growing loose. Dr Eric Budzislawski, the medical officer who examined her at the embassy, suspected liver trouble and advised further investigation, but she was too busy to return to the United States just yet. Italy's politics were still remarkably volatile.

At length, in the late autumn, Mrs Luce allowed friends to persuade her to consult specialists in the US Naval Hospital at Naples. She was hardly surprised or reassured when their investigations produced findings similar to those recorded in

New York. One consultant, however, seemed puzzled by the state of her mouth. He asked for a further specimen of urine for more intensive tests and insisted that whatever the political situation, it was vital she return to America for a rest. She therefore went home for Christmas and New Year, and almost at once began to feel better. Her appetite improved, the tiredness and irritability disappeared. It seemed Italy did not suit her constitution. It was as though there was something in the old warnings about the deadly Roman night air.

Once again, however, she was to have the serenity of a holiday shattered. Early in the New Year, while still luxuriating in the release from work and strain, she received a handwritten letter from Rome, from her Diplomatic Minister and Counsellor, Eldbridge Durbrow. Its contents were apparently too confidential to be trusted to even the most discreet stenographer or typist. An urgent message had been received from the US Naval Hospital, tests on Mrs Luce's urine specimen having revealed minute traces of arsenic. She should consult a toxicologist in New York immediately. Her story and clinical condition suggested that, somewhere in Rome, at the embassy or the Villa Taverna, or at some official function, she was being systematically poisoned by repeated tiny doses of arsenic. Durbrow advised her to contact the CIA forthwith.

Mrs Luce was startled to find that the CIA already knew and that she had unwittingly informed them herself. It was the ear, nose and throat consultant who had casually asked her whether any of her medicines contained arsenic, an occasional (although discredited) constituent of tonics. Out of amusement she mentioned this to a friend in the CIA before returning to the United States. He, in turn, worried and intrigued by the question, had made time on a routine trip to

Naples to check with the Naval Hospital, and found the doctors' assessment disquieting.

The ambassador, it seemed, presented a difficult problem of diagnosis. Her illness, though obviously troublesome, was remarkably intangible. The symptoms could not be precisely defined. She could not remember exactly when tiredness or irritability had first set in or when her legs had begun to ache. It was harder still for her to assess or explain to anyone else the exact severity of her various discomforts. The examination produced almost nothing to observe, except perhaps a little weight loss with mild anaemia: diffuse, non-specific findings which might arise from many different causes. Anaemia can itself, for instance, provoke a sense of physical weariness. With an individual like Clare Boothe Luce, exposed as she was to an exceptionally heavy burden of responsibility and a punishing work schedule, the temptation was to put the symptoms down to a reactive depression, an emotional exhaustion brought on by massive psychological pressures. It was the alert ear, nose and throat specialist, however, who, puzzled by a persistent catarrhal inflammation of nose and mouth, recalled clinical descriptions of that rare condition, chronic arsenic poisoning.

Arsenic taken in a large dose produces dramatic, well-recognized symptoms within the hour: abdominal pain, nausea, vomiting and diarrhoea, succeeded by prostration and collapse. Arsenic given in small repetitive doses, however, only produces rather ill-defined symptoms which appear gradually and may mimic those of any of a dozen naturally occurring diseases. The victim rather than collapsing fades gradually into ill-health, and during this slow deterioration the most difficult first step may be for it to occur to a doctor that his or her patient is being poisoned.

To heighten the predicament, the symptoms of chronic

arsenic poisoning are hardly remarkable. In the first phase, the patient complains of weakness and languor, loss of appetite with some nausea, occasional vomiting and a heaviness and discomfort in the stomach. Diarrhoea may also occur. As the symptoms worsen, there may be discomfort and redness of the eyes, similar to a mild conjunctivitis, and an annoying catarrh with sneezing and vocal hoarseness. Often a rash appears which may be hard to distinguish from a wide variety of other skin conditions. In cases where exposure has been prolonged, the hair as well as nails may become easily damaged and fall out.

More serious cases can lead to a jaundice following a swelling of the liver. The nervous system may also come under attack, with sharp headaches or evidence of damage to the nerves of the limbs: a polyneuritis which causes a disturbance of sensation and partial weakness, especially in legs and feet. Sometimes a muscular soreness means that pressure from bedclothes can be enough to cause discomfort, or there may be paraesthesia, a 'pins and needles' sensation, or even frank pain about the knee, ankle or foot. More often, however, there is a diminution in sensation, a numbness, a 'falling asleep' of legs and feet. With the strength of muscle groups impaired, there may be a definite weakening in such movements as drawing back the toes. Eventually, with continued poisoning, the patient may fall into an apathy degenerating slowly into semi-idiocy and eventually slipping thereafter inch by inch into death.

Arsenic has, throughout history, been a traditional tool of the poisoner. Colourless and tasteless as it is, it can be administered to an unsuspecting victim with ease. The resulting illness may even pass unrecognized, despite the attentions of doctors and specialists, and the victim fade and die with the cause wrongly diagnosed. But arsenic has one overriding disadvantage, a disadvantage so great that toxicologists have marvelled at anyone hazarding the gamble of using it as a poison: it leaves an invisible but indelible mark on its victims. The detection of arsenic poisoning becomes inevitable from the moment it is suspected. The poisoning may have ceased, or the victim have been long dead, yet every dose of arsenic swallowed can still be detected and measured. Deposited throughout the tissues and fluids, present in the hair and nails, it preserves a body from decay long after death. And the analysis of a single hair or a splinter of finger nail will still yield an accurate chronological account of the repeated chemical assaults made on the sufferer.

The naval hospital doctors had been only too aware of the implications behind their suspicions of arsenic poisoning in the case of Clare Boothe Luce. They had on their hands not only a possible assassination attempt to investigate but also the responsibility of safeguarding their ambassador from further danger. Mrs Luce's ambassadorship had hardly been marked by tranquillity. A list of potential assassins would not be difficult to compile, while the slightest hint of an investigation could provoke the wildest speculation and repercussion. Only suppose that the ambassador was being poisoned by one of her American staff, or that an Italian, of whatever political persuasion, was administering the arsenic. And should the would-be poisoner turn out to be a Communist, then the effects on public opinion in America and on the delicate balances in East–West relations might be unimaginable.

The physicians resolved their dilemma in the classically approved medical manner: they said nothing. Instead they insisted that Mrs Luce return to America for a complete rest and so quietly removed her from the danger zone. The vital specimen of urine, dispatched to the US Naval Medical

Center at Bethesda, was labelled as a sample from 'Seaman Jones'.

Mrs Luce found it almost impossible to credit the idea of someone trying to poison her, but then a toxicologist consulted in New York confirmed the findings of the specialists in Naples. As the top-secret panic got under way, Mrs Luce found herself being interrogated by two CIA agents who told her she had been swallowing small, less-than-lethal doses of arsenic over a considerable period. The poisoner, they explained, must be someone close enough to have repeated access to her food and drink. Until the poisoner was identified, it was common sense to suspect everyone in her household and at the embassy. She was especially shocked when one investigator, with logical reasonableness, took her aside to ask if she was having 'any difficulties' with her husband.

The CIA representative at the Rome embassy, faced with an overwhelming list of suspects, had in the meantime set his agents the undercover task of investigating the backgrounds of all those who handled or prepared food at the embassy or the Villa Taverna. He was particularly anxious to discover the political inclinations and connections of every one of the servants. He then began to concentrate on establishing up-to-date dossiers on all Americans in Rome.

Meanwhile the State Department ordered that Mrs Luce should stay in the United States until the mystery was solved. A team of experts was on its way to Italy. In Rome, it was almost casually announced that a firm of architects and engineers had been commissioned to prepare plans to remodel and modernize both the Villa Taverna and parts of the embassy. Experts would be arriving to make preliminary studies and were expected to spend a week or so observing domestic routines in each establishment. These investigations would cover every aspect of housekeeping, from the selection and ordering of supplies to the preparation and serving of meals and drinks. Staff were asked to co-operate.

With this licence to intrude unobtrusively, the investigators delved into the most minute details, identifying everyone with any access to the food placed before the ambassador, from the chef who masterminded the banquets to the servant who modestly prepared a plate of late-night sandwiches. Within days, however, it dawned that it was going to be extremely difficult for even an army of top-rank investigators to detect a poisoner while the intended victim was absent and no poison was being administered. Tentatively, it was suggested that Mrs Luce might return to Rome to act as decoy. The State Department curtly vetoed the experiment.

Finally, convinced that there was nothing to be discovered at the embassy, the team concentrated on the Villa Taverna. The small, repetitive doses suggested a poisoner with a close and prolonged association, even an intimate acquaintance with the ambassador. Accordingly, they concentrated on the private apartments, and it was here that the clue finally emerged when an observant agent noticed an accumulation of grey dust on a black disc which lay exposed on the Linguaphone machine in the study-bedroom. Even as he inspected it, a maid arrived with dusters and mops. Yes, she confirmed, although the ambassador was away, the room was cleaned each day, and certainly the Linguaphone was dusted. Since the room was not in use, the windows were kept shut.

A remarkable quantity of dust therefore seemed to be accumulating in a room that was closed and unoccupied. The agent paused to watch the maid's routine, and next morning returned to the study early, before the maid arrived. Again a film of greyish-white dust lay on the black Linguaphone record, and this time the agent brushed it up carefully into an envelope. A wider search revealed accumulations of the same dust trapped in the folds of the draperies and miniature lodes of greyish-white powder gathered in corners and crevices and even spread thin on the surfaces of cosmetics. All at once the investigator remembered Mrs Luce's complaints not only about bitter breakfast coffee but also about the way her record player repeatedly broke down, its mechanism strangely clogged with accumulations of dust.

The laboratory report on the dust from the record showed it to consist of a fine powder containing minute flakes of paint, its chemical analysis revealing a high concentration of lead arsenate. The investigators found themselves gazing up in surmise at the intricately painted study ceiling, that perfect example of Italian Renaissance décor which had so entranced a succession of American ambassadors. Could this be the source of the trouble? Yes, indeed, flakes of paint taken from its florid rosettes and its finely moulded entwining branches and leaves turned out to be heavy with lead arsenate. The unique chain suspension of the ceiling was recalled, as were Mrs Luce's grumbles about the disturbance caused by even the footsteps of servants on the floor above. More disquietingly, the agents grew aware of the mechanical juddering of the American washing-machine immediately overhead.

Arsenic was no longer legal as a constituent of paint. Inorganic compounds of arsenic had once been widely used as pigments, and one particular compound, Scheele's green or cupric arsenate, enjoyed such a vogue that its method of manufacture was kept a closely guarded secret until a process for preparing it was devised and published by Liebig in 1822. Because of its poisonous nature, however, manufacturers in different countries gave it different names in the hope of selling it as innocuous. As a further disguise, they mixed it with baryta and gypsum to lighten the colour. Thus it accumulated a variety of aliases: Paris green, French green, Vienna green, Mitis green, Schweinfurth green, emerald green. Despite such subterfuges, the hazards associated with the use of arsenical pigments were by the turn of the century fully recognized. By the late 1920s and early 1930s, their use was controlled by legislation.

A small, independent decorator, Nicolo Pacella, readily agreed on questioning that he had been responsible for decorating the ambassador's study. This work had been carried out three years before, in 1951, though on that occasion he simply retouched the walls with distemper. He was certain the distemper contained no poisonous substances and was absolutely harmless. So far as he was aware, the last substantial decoration of the study took place in 1922. The ceiling itself had certainly not been touched since. The case looked to be complete.

Cushny's great *Textbook of Pharmacology and Therapeutics* (1899) remarks:

> The milder symptoms [of chronic arsenic poisoning] may arise from its therapeutic use, but typical cases are generally due to the presence of arsenic in the form of dyes in wall paper, carpets or clothes, or in stuffed animals in the rooms inhabited by the victims . . . it often seems to be inhaled in the form of fine dust, which falls from the walls or other objects.

In the late nineteenth century, such accidental arsenical poisoning was considered usual enough for the Medical Society in London to set up a committee to consider the matter. In about 1880 the committee issued a list of items in which arsenical pigments were commonly used. These included coloured papers, playing cards, Christmas tree decorations, wrappers for sweetmeats, fabrics for curtains and furniture coverings, carpets and linoleum, American cloth, printed table baizes, venetian blinds, coloured soaps, indiarubber balls and distemper.

In 1923, a commission set up to investigate arsenical 'house-poisoning' in Sweden decided that it must be demonstrated, among other things, that the symptoms commenced within one to three months of the start of exposure and disappeared within three months of it ceasing. The commission was rigorous in its approach, accepting only a few of the ninety-one cases referred to it by Swedish doctors. Nevertheless, in a wide review of international medical literature, it discovered 125 case-reports of arsenical house-poisoning, sixty-one of which fulfilled its own criteria. The Swedish commission found that the symptoms differed greatly according to how the arsenic was absorbed. Where the arsenic was thought to be inhaled as a dust or even a gas, the principal symptoms were lassitude, headache, giddiness and irritation of the eyes and throat. If the arsenic was actually swallowed, such digestive disturbances as diarrhoea were usual. In neither case, however, was polyneuritis an especially common symptom.

Yet Clare Boothe Luce, exposed to lead arsenate, had suffered a definite polyneuritis, with numbness and heaviness of the right foot. This seemed to be a characteristic symptom of lead arsenate poisoning in particular. In 1941, in an apple-growing district of the United States, following extensive spraying of orchards with lead arsenate, several workers were found to have arsenic in their urine with polyneuritis a common effect. An editorial in the *Lancet* attributed both Mrs Luce's anaemia and her polyneuritis to the lead component in the dust from the study ceiling at the Villa Taverna.

The ceiling was duly stripped of its old paint, the entire study redecorated. The 'planned alterations' to embassy and official residence were quietly shelved. The agents returned home. Clare Boothe Luce resumed her duties in Rome and the incident was considered closed.

And so it might have remained indefinitely but for a misunderstanding with a presidential press secretary. In 1956, Eisenhower was re-elected to the White House for a second term. At this natural pause in his administration, Clare Boothe Luce asked to be replaced. She had served nearly four years in one of the most arduous of diplomatic postings. She had negotiated with eight successive Italian governments. Her efforts had contributed to the resolution of the Trieste crisis, and she had helped to shift Italian public opinion away from hostility to the United States towards an atmosphere of goodwill and friendship.

In explaining her resignation to the President, Mrs Luce recounted the episode of chronic arsenic poisoning, mentioning that she felt tired and that she now had fresh problems with her health. The presidential press secretary, in announcing her retirement, then unexpectedly let slip the story of the poisonous ceiling, so publicizing an incident that had been kept a close secret for nearly eighteen months. It caught the imagination of the press and appeared on the front pages of newspapers throughout Europe and America. In the Luce household, consternation reigned. Henry had, as proprietor of the influential trio of *Time*, *Life* and *Fortune* magazines, conscientiously maintained the secrecy only to find himself now being scooped by rivals.

In Rome, the foreign correspondents indulged in some private sleuthing, yet the staff of the Villa Taverna seemed surprisingly unaware of the episode while all the paint manufacturers insisted that the story was impossible since paint no longer contained arsenic. Eminent Italian physicians consulted by the press were also inclined to be sceptical. One or two had heard of arsenic house-poisoning, though they had no experience of the condition. Right-wing opinion in Italy viewed the story as a diplomatic version of an abortive Communist attempt to poison the ambassador, while a left-wing newspaper claimed to have information that the arsenic came from a special tonic which Mrs Luce was supposedly taking to restore her youth.

In the United States, the story was greeted with a similar incredulity and Clare Boothe Luce, who once waspishly declared that the columnist Dorothy Thompson was 'the only woman who ever conducted her menopause in public', found herself accused of having suffered nothing more serious than hot flushes. To all the commentators, the story looked too neat, too much like one that Clare Boothe Luce might have invented about herself. Many distinguished medical authorities consulted by the press seemed unaware of the known cases of house-poisoning which had occurred during the lifetime of their professional predecessors or of the circumstances which had led to the introduction in practically every country of legislation which banned the use of arsenic in paint or articles intended for domestic use. They were disinclined to accept the tale of dust from a painted ceiling poisoning an ambassador as even an interesting anachronism, an example of a twentieth-century woman falling victim to a nineteenth-century disorder. They were moreover apparently unaware of the continuing steady trickle of case-reports of illness occurring in individuals accidentally exposed to various sprays and dusts containing inorganic arsenical compounds.

It can be the fate of politicians and diplomats to face trial by public opinion. The newspapers found it hard to accept the idea of house-poisoning. The story of Clare Boothe Luce and the poisonous Renaissance ceiling was judged by the press and found wanting. Although it was not immediately apparent, it marked the start of her career's decline. As her biographer, Wilfred Sheed, has pointed out, the incident did contain its wryly humorous side. For years the husband and wife team of Clare Boothe and Henry Luce, she with her acid wit and he with his publishing empire, had been surreptitiously dubbed 'Arsenic and Old Luce'.

Chapter 7

The Visitor from a Far Country

The Shotley peninsula lies on the edge of Suffolk between the tidal mudflats of the estuaries of the rivers Orwell and Stour. At its tip the naval barracks at Shotley Gate face, across the waters to the south, Parkestone Quay, and to the east the port of Felixstowe. On its northern margin the Orwell carries shipping upriver to Ipswich docks. The peninsula itself consists of a gently undulating countryside with remote, scattered communities of villages that are still, today, much as they were before the First World War, except that the rural poverty of the earlier years of this century has long since lost its grip.

About five miles south of Ipswich, within the parish of Freston, Latimer Cottages stand at the roadside in a position of isolation from other dwellings. In 1910 the cottages were divided into a row of three homesteads, and in the middle cottage lived a farmworker, Mr George Chapman, with his wife Frances and four of her children from a previous marriage. Mr Chapman had only lately moved from Ipswich with his step-family, and the two younger girls, Annie Goodall, aged nine, and her sister Emily, aged seven, were attending Freston village school.

On 13 September 1910, Annie Goodall was overtaken at school by a sudden attack of vomiting. When the family doctor, Dr Carey, from the neighbouring village of Holbrook, visited her next day, he found her running a fever, with her temperature standing at 105°F. Within twenty-four hours she was showing signs of an inflammation of the lungs, having been delirious during the night, and on the third night of her illness she suffered from vomiting and diarrhoea. The next day she died. A classmate who delivered a wreath from the village school to her home was shown Annie lying in her coffin. She kissed her farewell, and Mrs Chapman remarked on how her daughter had changed colour since being put in the coffin that morning, her lips having turned quite blue. It is said that four little girls drew Annie on a bier to her burial, which took place in Freston churchyard on the 20th. The day after the funeral Mrs Chapman complained of headache and feeling sick.

When once again sent for on the afternoon of the 22nd, Dr Carey found Mrs Chapman requesting medicine and very poorly. Her temperature was high, her breathing quite rapid, and her lungs already showed a degree of congestion. A neighbour from up the road, Mrs Parker from Turkey Farm, kindly offered to help with nursing the invalid through the night, but when Dr Carey called again at ten o'clock the next morning, he discovered his patient almost pulseless and gasping for breath. Highly concerned by the startling speed of Mrs Chapman's decline, he promptly sought a second opinion from a colleague, Dr Herbert Brown of Ipswich. Dr Brown arrived at Latimer Cottages by twelve noon, too late to find Mrs Chapman alive, though he was able to obtain and take away a sample of sputum. This he described as 'brownish in colour, as though tinged with anchovy sauce, and did not at all resemble ordinary pneumonic sputum'. Nevertheless, when submitted for analysis, the specimen showed up nothing unusual besides the germs normally present in a case of pneumonia.

Mr George Chapman rose at his usual time on the morning of his wife's funeral, 26 September, and left the house to go to work, though he did complain of backache and 'feeling bad'. He attended the funeral later, then went home to bed. Meanwhile, at Turkey Farm on the same day, Mrs Parker was also taken ill. The local doctors were by now fully aware of having something out of the way and rapidly lethal on their doorsteps, and Dr H. P. Sleigh, the Medical Officer of Health for the local authority, the Rural District of Samford, was also called into consultation. Blood samples were taken from Mr Chapman, and a specimen of fluid was obtained from Mrs Parker's lung. These specimens were sent for investigation to Dr Llewellyn Heath, bacteriologist at the East Suffolk and Ipswich Hospital. On the 29th, before Dr Heath had a chance to come forward with any definite findings, both patients died, Mrs Parker during the morning and Mr Chapman that afternoon.

According to a report in the *East Anglian Daily Times* of 5 October 1910, Dr Heath's analysis in fact revealed a 'disease suspected to be a highly infectious and fatal one, which fortunately very seldom occurs'. The funerals of both Mrs Parker and Mr Chapman had been held in haste on the day following their deaths. The undertakers were not even given time to screw Mr Chapman's nameplate on to his coffin lid and the rector held the services in the open air, those attending having their clothes disinfected afterwards. All bedding and linen, clothes, curtains and furnishings from the homes of the victims were either burnt or disinfected, while the rooms were thoroughly fumigated. Quicklime was spread over their cottage gardens and the surviving members of their families were forbidden to enter their homes but were placed in isolation in the local workhouse.

Another of Mrs Chapman's daughters, Edith, had as a fourteen-year-old been working in service at Freston rectory during the daytime. As an old lady she remembered how those days had been a dreadful time for them, 'me being the eldest at home' and 'we . . . at the mercy of the world as they burnt our home and we only had our clothes we wore when they took us and the other family for isolation to Tattingstone Workhouse'.

There they remained for three weeks, shocked and bewildered by the short, sharp tragedy that had struck out so murderously at their families. Nevertheless, the *East Anglian Daily Times* was able in its report to reassure readers that the precautions taken, together with the absence of any fresh cases, indicated that the danger of a recurrence of the disease should by now be safely passing. Edith would always remember how, just before the outbreak which killed her sister, mother and stepfather, Mr Chapman brought home a rabbit caught for the family dinner. Fifty-nine years later she wrote she had never been able to eat rabbit since.

The reason for the speed at which the last two funerals were held in fact lay in an urgent memorandum from Dr Llewellyn Heath to Dr Sleigh, dated 30 September: 'I found this morning and last night the B. pestis in cultures of the blood made from Brown's punctures.' It was on the basis of this discovery of the plague germ, *Pasteurella pestis*, that immediate recommendations were made for the house contents to be burnt, all contacts isolated, the infection hospital opened and compensation paid for property destroyed. Dr Heath also wrote that, 'I thought it better to have a big name at the back of me if necessary', and this was why, on the same

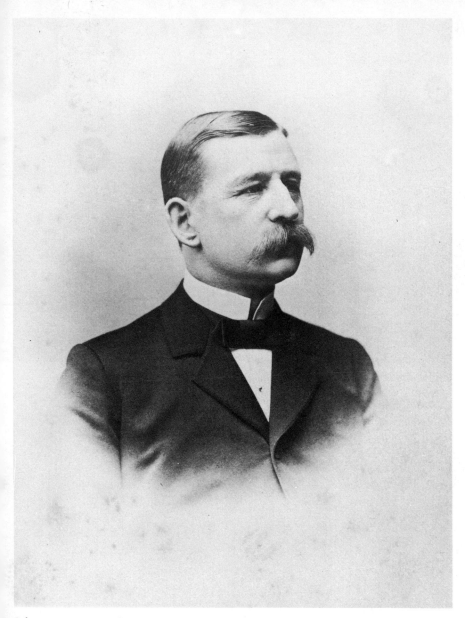

Salomon August Andrée, the leader of the Swedish balloon expedition

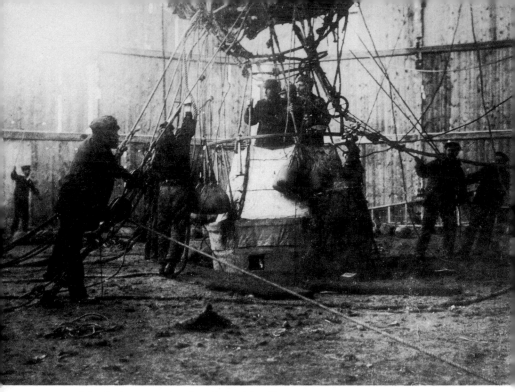

The *Eagle* prepared and ready for lift-off

The shore watchers' last view of the *Eagle*

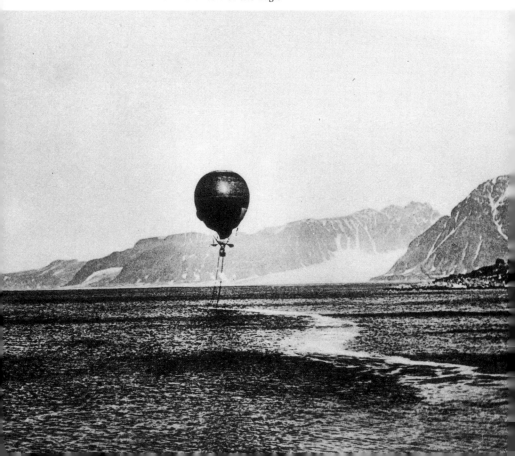

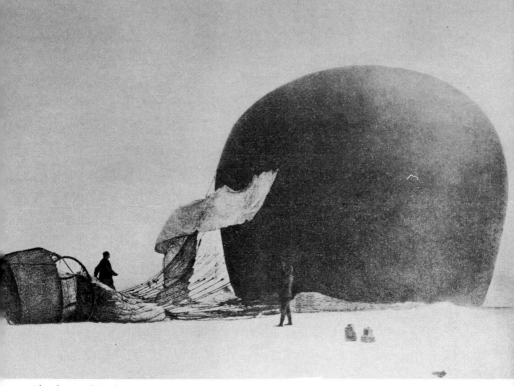

The doomed *Eagle* stranded on the ice

The explorers manhandle their boat on the pack-ice

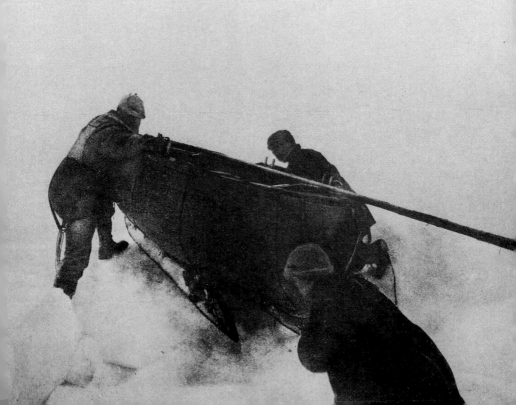

Strindberg and Fraenkel survey 'a welcome kill'

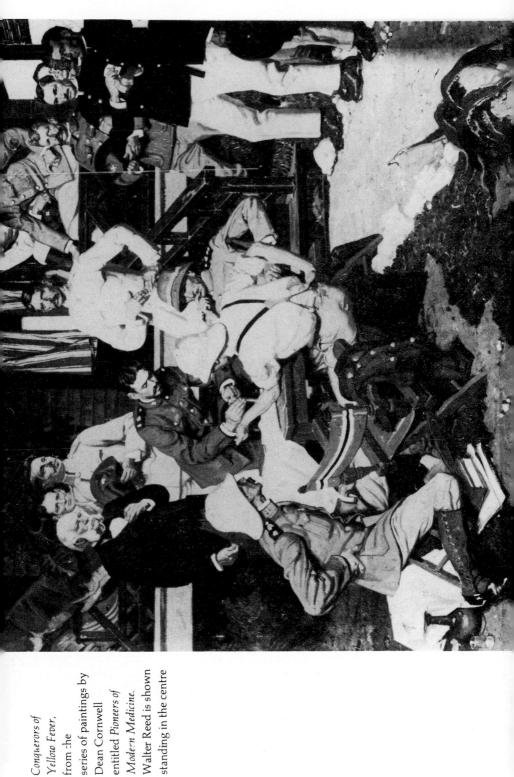

Conquerors of Yellow Fever, from the series of paintings by Dean Cornwell entitled *Pioneers of Modern Medicine*. Walter Reed is shown standing in the centre

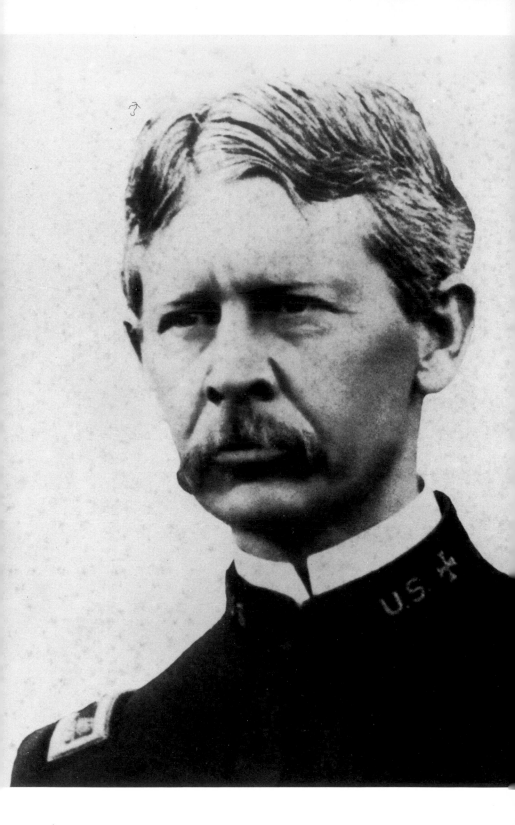

WAR DEPARTMENT,
SURGEON GENERAL'S OFFICE,
WASHINGTON.

(OVER) Sept. 7. 1900
1.15 P.M.

My dear Carroll:

Hip! Hip! Hurrah! God be praised for the news from Cuba today — Carroll much improved — Prognosis very good"! I shall simply go out and get boiling drunk! Really I can never recall such a sense of relief in all my life, as the news of your recovery gives me! And then, too, would you believe it? The Typhoid Report is on its way to the Upper Office!

Well, I'm damned if I don't get drunk twice !!!

(OVER) God bless you, my boy.

Affectionately,
Reed

Come home as soon as you can & see your wife & babies

Did the Mosquito do it?

The letter, dated 7 September 1900, which Reed wrote to James Carroll to congratulate him on his recovery

left Major Walter Reed

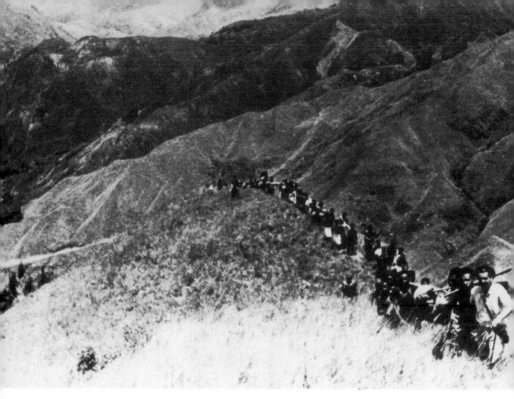

A kuru patrol in the country of the North Fore Indians, Papua New Guinea. The photograph illustrates the area's geographical difficulties of communication

A vine suspension bridge built to ease the progress of kuru patrols in the Fore country

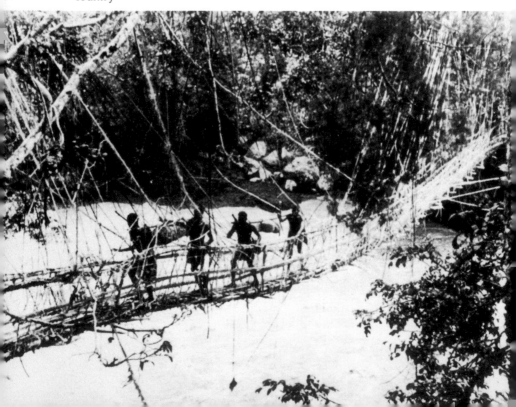

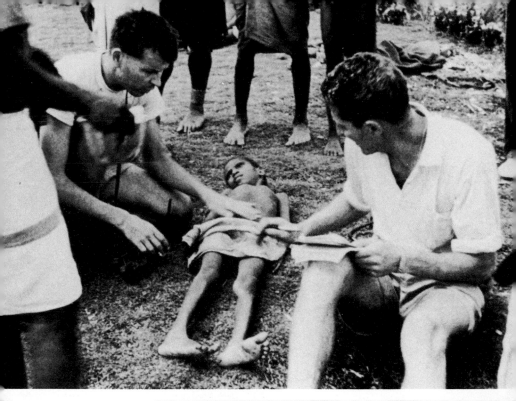

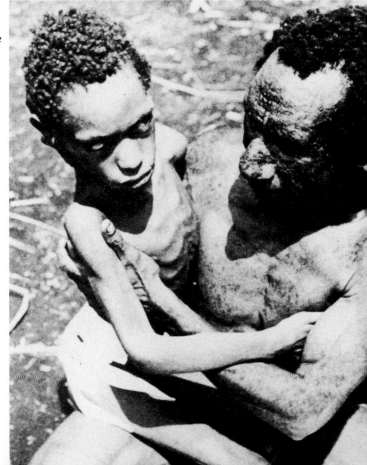

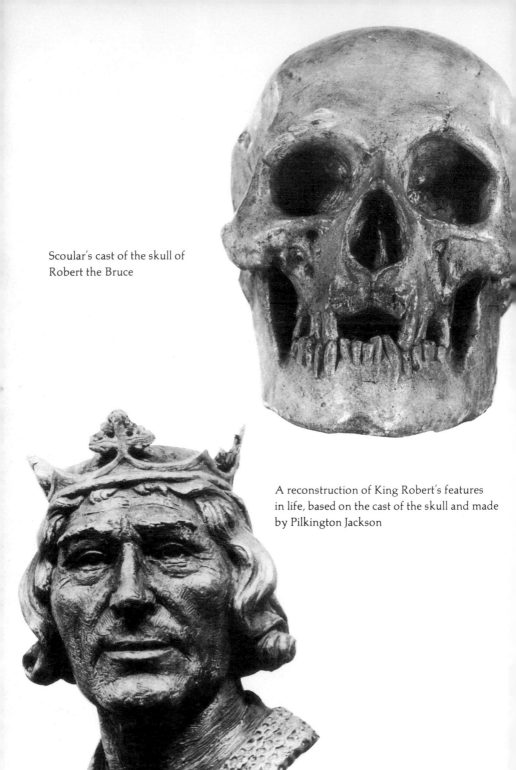

Scoular's cast of the skull of Robert the Bruce

A reconstruction of King Robert's features in life, based on the cast of the skull and made by Pilkington Jackson

opposite Dr Vilhelm Møller-Christensen excavates a medieval leper graveyard

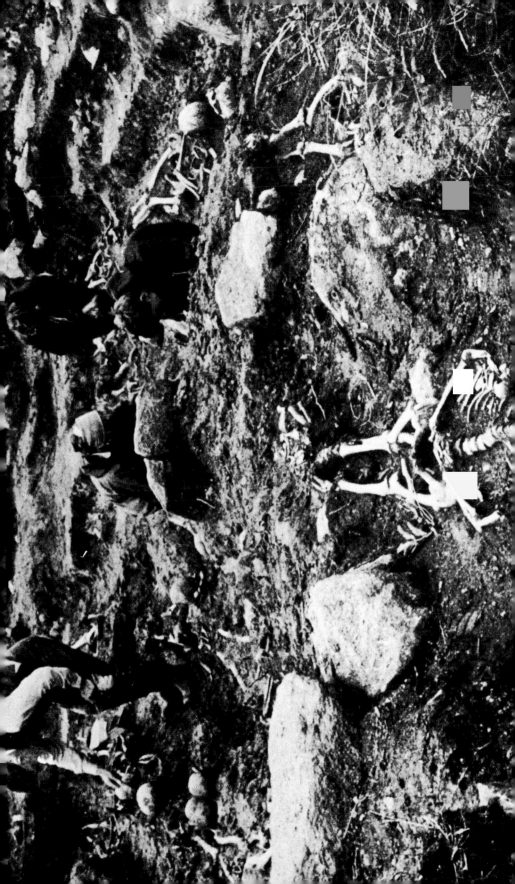

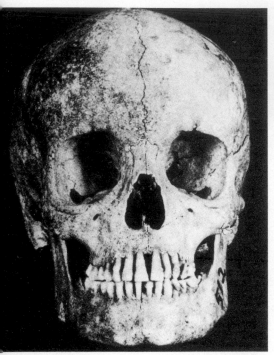

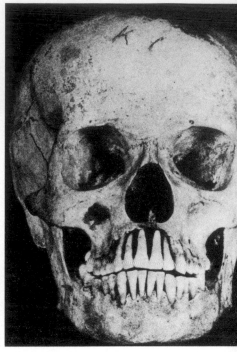

A sequence of skulls showing
the progressive stages of the changes which
leprosy may cause to the upper jaw

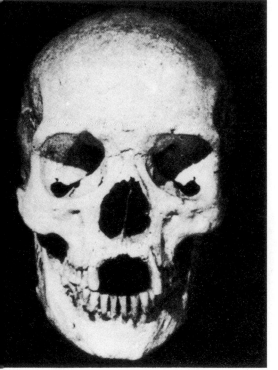

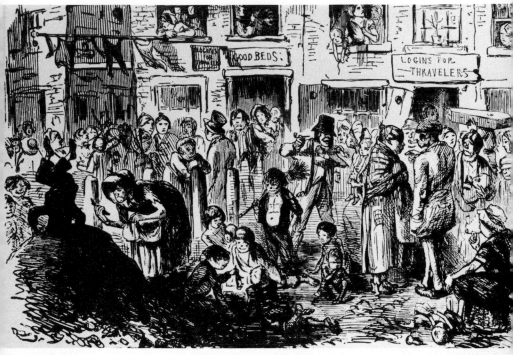

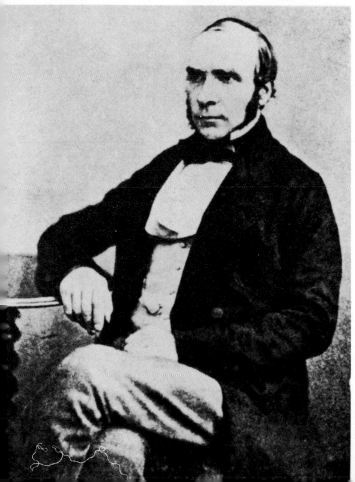

Dr John Snow

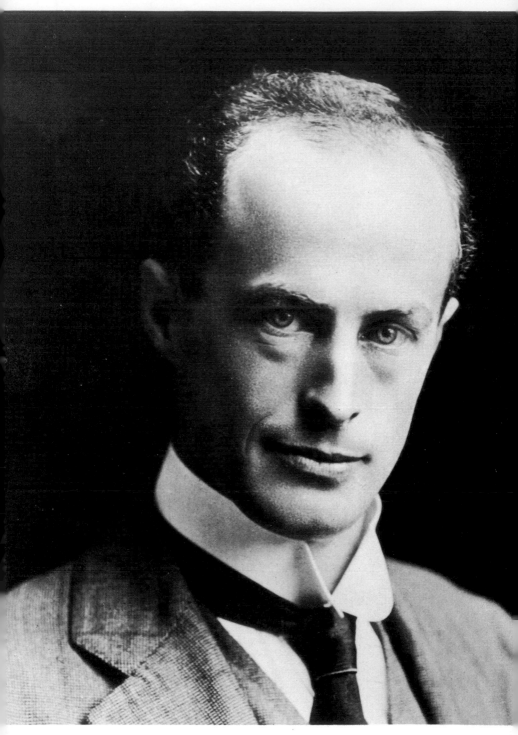

Portrait photograph of Sir Douglas Mawson, taken in 1911 before he departed for Antarctica

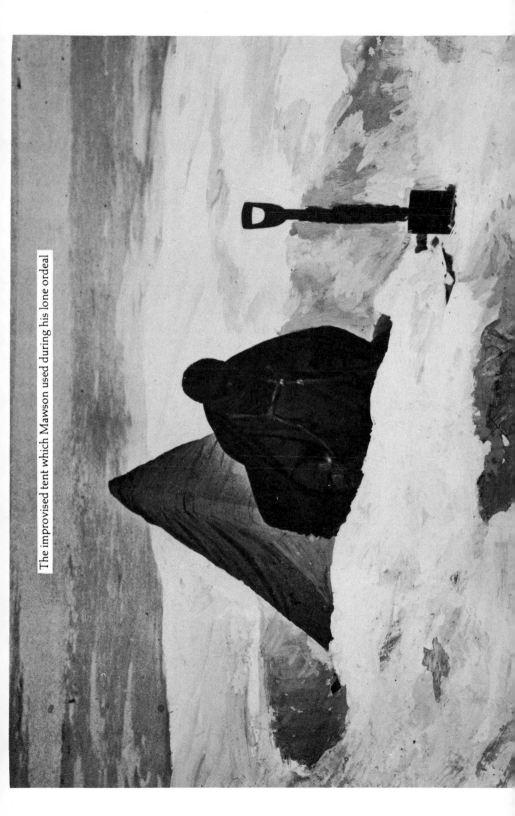

The improvised tent which Mawson used during his lone ordeal

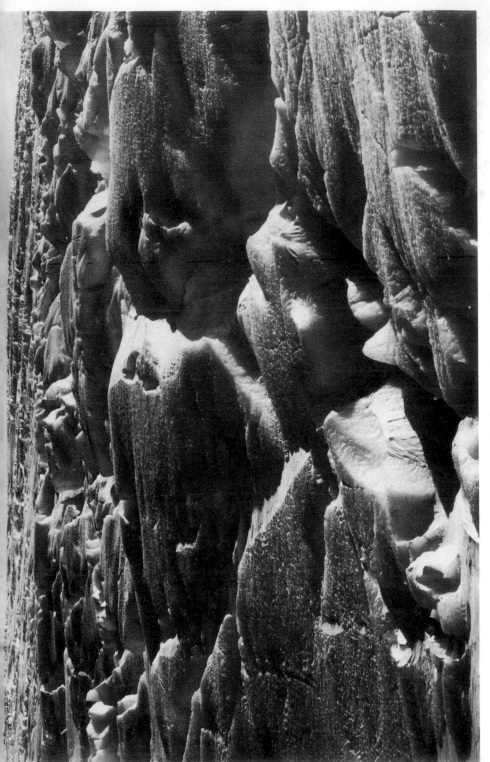

Terrain of the kind faced by the Australian Antarctic Expedition of 1911–14:

day, he travelled to Cambridge to visit Sims Woodhead, the Professor of Pathology to the University. Early that evening a telegram delivered to Dr Sleigh confirmed Professor Woodhead's agreement that the plague bacillus was present in the specimens. Plague, the personification of death reaping with a scythe for earlier generations of Europeans, was thought in the popular imagination to belong firmly with history. Yet here it had reappeared, raising its grisly head in a quiet corner of the English county of Suffolk during the first decade of the twentieth century.

Historically speaking, plague is indeed among the best-documented of diseases, having been, for humankind, a periodically occurring large-scale disaster. It may be open to speculation that it was an epidemic of plague which Jehovah marshalled against the Philistines after they stole the Ark of the Covenant (I Samuel 5–6), when 'the hand of the Lord was against the city with a very great destruction: and he smote the men of the city, both small and great, and they had emerods in their secret parts'. It is virtually certain that it was a pandemic of plague which, in AD 542–3, reached Europe through Rome out of Egypt during Justinian's reign. The Black Death, which swept like an invisible, malevolent tidal wave across Europe between 1346 and 1349, arriving in Britain in 1348, was fully documented in contemporary writings, and as it cut down the lives of about half the population it seemed a fulfilment of the visionary prophecies of disaster in the Book of Revelation that foretold the end of the world. The plague symptoms were graphically described, both in their bubonic form, where agonizing swellings or buboes appeared as lymph glands came to be infected in the groin, armpit or neck, and in their pneumonic form, where the lungs were inflamed and the victims became in turn highly infectious. While the chances of surviving plague in its bubonic form stood at less than 50 per cent, death was a certainty, usually within three to four days, where there was a pneumonic infection. The descriptive term 'Black Death' is thought to have arisen in part from the fact that bubonic plague caused dark patches of bleeding into the skin, but also from the tendency of those slain by pneumonic plague to turn slatey blue after dying. (Edith Goodall witnessed how the body of her mother, Mrs Chapman, became black and swollen in death.)

The Black Death established plague as an endemic hazard in Europe for the best part of three centuries. It continued to flare up sporadically, especially in crowded cities in warm summer weather, but the Great Plague of 1665 was its closing, most flamboyant gesture. For reasons still not fully understood, the germ then seemed to lose its virulence and to die out from Western Europe. However, by the 1890s medical officers who saw service abroad in India and the Far East in the British Empire found themselves becoming acquainted with cases of plague at first hand. This time the source lay with an epidemic which slowly developed into a pandemic after having its origins in the 1850s when refugees spread the disease during a rebellion in Yunnan province in China. As a result, in the summer of 1894, 100,000 citizens of Canton died of plague, terrified survivors then carrying the infection to the China ports, including Hong Kong. From there it rapidly made its way to Bombay and Calcutta, often officially denied but accounting for appalling death-rates among Indians in both towns and villages. It spread in due course to the western ports of North and South America, setting off an epidemic in which 122 died in 1903–4 in California, and also reaching Australia among other locations.

In Britain, with its world-wide empire trade, the authorities were well aware of the threat which plague could pose in one port or another at any time. It came ashore in Glasgow in the summer of 1900, and killed sixteen people. The incident prompted the Medical Department of the Local Government Board to issue in September 1900 a 'Plague Memorandum' to local medical officers of health, which stated:

Plague having for the space of nearly two centuries receded from Europe, has in recent years once more trended westward, and has now again appeared in Great Britain. Sanitary Authorities of England and Wales will therefore need to be on the alert to detect the presence of this disease in their districts, with a view to prevent its becoming epidemic among their populations.

It was not felt that plague would 'readily fasten on that section of our population which is properly housed, cleanly, and generally, in a sanitary sense, well to do'. The more direct threat lay with the danger that the disease might gain a foothold in 'insanitary areas such as are peopled by the poorest class, and where overcrowding of persons in houses and dirt and squalor of dwellings and of inhabitants tend to prevail'.

The memorandum then set out the precautions which should be taken with notifying outbreaks, isolating contacts, protecting medical workers with inoculations of Haffkine's plague prophylactic, developed during the epidemics in India, caring for the sick, and disinfecting all articles and living accommodation. It also included a description of the symptoms expected to occur in different types of plague. The association of rodents, especially of rats, with plague was well established in the folklore of all peoples who had suffered its onslaught, and the memorandum acknowledged this association when it commented:

Plague affects rats as well as the human subject; it may, indeed, be found causing mortality among these lower animals antecedent to its definite invasion of the population. There can be no doubt that the rat and man are, as regards plague, reciprocally infective.

Yet the correlation of rats with plague was still not as yet universally accepted by the scientific community. The identification of the plague bacillus itself had been made only six years earlier, in the plague hospitals of Hong Kong in 1894, though a controversy raged for years over whether its discoverer had been Dr Kitasato, a distinguished Japanese microbiologist, or Alexandre Yersin, a Swiss explorer and doctor. Then a remarkable piece of research was published in the *Annales de L'Institut Pasteur* in October 1898. The author was Dr Paul Louis Simmond, who while working in Indo-China and Bombay had been struck by his observation that a dramatic mortality among rats did indeed herald outbreaks among humans. Working in a tent through the Indian monsoon, Dr Simmond found that the digestive tracts of rat fleas taken from infected rats also contained the plague organism. To this he added the highly important discovery that human plague victims carried detectable flea bites and that, contrary to the orthodox medical view, rat fleas would bite man. It was the rat fleas passing from dead or dying to healthy animals which saw to the transmission of plague and hence which passed it on to human hosts.

Dr Simmond's notions were initially held up to ridicule. The Indian Plague Commission continued to feel in 1899 that there was 'absolutely no evidence that the disease has ever been carried from one country to another by plague infected rats in ships'. In 1902, an editorial in the *Indian Medical Gazette* dismissed Simmond's ideas as being 'worthless' and 'completely demolished' by other research. The new Indian Plague Commission, however, which started work in Bombay in 1905, took an altogether more open-minded attitude. Its report was published in 1908, and, while it gave scant credit to Simmond's ideas, it also, in effect, confirmed and augmented each of his findings and deductions in practically every detail. Simmond stood vindicated, and though a further period passed before his work was properly acknowledged, the unholy triad of rat, rat flea and plague bacillus became from then on fully accepted as the cause of the spread and transmission of plague.

In Suffolk, on 1 October 1910, Dr Sleigh, acting as local medical officer of health for Samford Rural District, gave notice of the positive diagnosis of plague made from the specimens taken from Mr Chapman and Mrs Parker to the Local Government Board in London. The board's inspector, the resonantly named Dr Timbrell Bulstrode, decided to visit Suffolk to make his own inquiries, and travelled down on the 4th. He asked that the specimens be sent on from Professor Woodhead for further investigation by the board's bacteriological adviser at the Lister Institute. Time had gone by, however, and the adviser could only work with 'such material as then remained'. It was perhaps not surprising that his search for pestis should, as he reported on 8 October, prove negative.

Dr Bulstrode made it clear that the matter would not be allowed to rest at this point, and meanwhile the board's adviser proceeded to an investigation of the bodies of a rat and a hare, both from near Freston. On the 12th he reached his conclusion: both were infected with *Pasteurella pestis*. Later checks on other rodent specimens from the area produced the same finding. The diagnosis of plague in the case of the human victims may still have retained a controversial shade. What was undeniable was that an epizootic of plague was in progress among the rodent population of the Shotley peninsula, and that these stricken animals represented a threat to human health. The implication was obvious: that the disease must have been brought ashore by rats from ships navigating the Orwell estuary.

A three-fold objective was now kept in view by Dr Bulstrode. First, the local population needed to be warned about the dangers of having any contact with dead or dying wild animals, and second a rigorous campaign should be mounted to strike at the rat population. Finally, local medical records should be scanned to see if any previous incidents of sudden acute illness might be attributed to unrecognized plague cases.

A special meeting of the Samford Rural District Council, held on 20 October, agreed to the printing and distribution of warning handbills and to the appointment of ratcatchers. The council blenched, however, at the idea of standing the expense of supplying rat poison. The chairman of the council made his views on this subject clear in a letter to Dr Sleigh:

> As to your suggestions . . . about killing rats, it seemed to us that you were not aware that nearly all farmers and householders carry on an incessant warfare with these animals but have to confess themselves beaten . . . Of course if the council offered to supply, free of cost, virus or poisons, large quantities would be applied for but for the most part it would be used only as a substitute for poisons which farmers and others would in the ordinary course pay for themselves.

The next day, when Dr Herbert Brown read of the council's decision in the *East Anglian Daily Times*, he at once wrote to Dr Sleigh expressing his indignation:

> It is quite obvious that they entirely fail to grasp the seriousness of the matter, and I think the Council have clearly shewn their hopeless incapacity and foolishness. If an epidemic spread they will

be responsible for it. Something ought to be done to bring this home
to them.

Yet over the course of the next week the sense of urgency
heightened, and on the 27th a joint committee of the district
council and Ipswich Corporation was set up, 'with full power
to take such steps as they should consider advisable'. Costs
were to be shared equally between the two authorities.

Schoolchildren were warned not to touch any corpses of
animals found in the countryside and landowners asked their
gamekeepers to watch for signs of rat mortality on their
estates. Circulated notices contained stern warnings against
handling or eating rabbits or hares, but even so a large
quantity of rabbits shot and buried in a pit at Wolverston, the
next village to Freston, was mysteriously spirited away
overnight. The systematic destruction of rats got under way
as farmers held ferreting parties and ratcatchers went to work.
The *Daily Mail*'s special correspondent sent in the following
description from Holbrook:

Along the hedge-bank an old man crept slowly. A small canvas
bag swung in one hand and he carried a spoon bound to the end of
a 3-ft stick in the other. Every now and then, at spots a few paces
apart, he shovelled a spoonful of white powder from a bag into the
bank and chuckled. 'That'll feed 'em,' he said to me in the broad
accents of Suffolk. 'They'll have it tonight, and when tomorrow they
come for it they'll find it ain't the same, and they'll just lay 'em
down and die.'

This old man in his corduroys and leggings, with his bag and his
spoon, is one of the veterans enlisted in the war against the rats in
the Orwell peninsula.

There were twenty ratcatchers operating, but not one of
them could be persuaded by the *Mail*'s correspondent to give
away the secret of his personal formula, deadly to all rats.

Meanwhile, in Felixstowe on 1 November, the town corporation instituted a rat cart to which, as it went its rounds,
householders could bring out their dead rats to be dipped in
disinfectant before being carried away for cremation. It was
estimated that between 6,000 and 8,000 rats were by now
dying each day on the peninsula itself.

As the war against the rats continued, Dr Bulstrode focused
attention on two other outbreaks of illness which fell under
suspicion of having been cases of plague. The first had
occurred between December 1906 and January 1907 at Charity
Farm Cottages in the eastern part of the peninsula, not far
north of Shotley. The cottages looked out across the estuary
and had a good view of Butterman's Bay, where ocean-going
ships, including many grain ships from international foreign
ports, would pause at anchor to lighten their loads by
transferring some of their cargo on to barges before proceeding upstream to Ipswich docks. The families involved at
Charity Farm had been Dr Carey's patients, and the death-
roll had risen to six after an acute pneumonia struck down in
quick succession a middle-aged woman, her married daughter who came to nurse her, a neighbour who came to nurse
the daughter, the neighbour's husband and son, and finally
her mother, who travelled down from Saxmundham to care
for the invalids. One further member of each family also
caught the disease but managed to rally and recover. The less
lucky ones had all been dead within two to five days of falling
ill.

The second suspicious example was more recent and had
caught up seven members of the same family, three of whom
recovered, between December 1909 and January 1910. This
time, however, the location lay outside the peninsula in the
hamlet of Trimley Lower Street on the north bank of the River
Orwell. There had been an inquest, since it occurred to the

family doctor that poisoning might be involved, the disease having made its attack so suddenly. One of the survivors, Honora Rouse, told the story of what befell her family in a deposition to the coroner, dated 5 February 1910:

There was my father and mother, myself and two sisters, Carrie and Alice, and two boys, Willie and John. On Sunday December 19th my mother had a headache when she awoke. She got up about 10 o'clock and was sick. She had sickness and diarrhoea and got worse and on Wednesday 22nd she went to bed about 4.30 p.m. – I went upstairs with her and helped her into bed. I went downstairs and at about 5 p.m. I went up again and found she was dead . . . On Sunday [26th] my sister Carrie turned up ill, and she and Willie were both full of sores, and Carrie had a knot on her neck. My mother had a knot on her neck while she was ill. Dr Hart was sent for on 2nd January, he came and attended her and she died on 5th January and on this day Alice fell ill. She was ill in the same way as the others, and had a knot and she died on the 10th January. My father also fell ill on 8th January. He was sick and had diarrhoea like the others but had a knot swell up on his thigh. He was removed to Ipswich Hospital on the 10th January. On the 11th January my two brothers, Willie and John, were taken to Barham Workhouse. On the Sunday following I heard that Willie was ill and I went to Barham and saw him. He had the same symptoms as the others and had a knot on his neck. He died on the 17th January – On the 22nd January I fell ill and went to the hospital and remained there till the 3rd February. I was ill in the same way as the others and had spots on my legs and also a knot inside my thigh and my face and arms were swollen. My brother John was also taken to the hospital and is still there.

The eighteen-year-old Honora, with her six-year-old brother John and their father, survived the assault of what Dr Bulstrode accepted as having been plague in its bubonic form. The earlier attack at Charity Farm Cottages he interpreted as another pneumonic example. It was impossible for any decisive proof or confirmation to emerge at this late stage, yet the evidence, on its circumstantial basis, looked strong. In the meantime the work on the destruction and examination of rats went on into 1911, though Dr Bulstrode died suddenly that July. A much-circulated local tradition that he died from plague was based on nothing but whimsy.

As part of the Local Government Board's investigations, an interesting piece of research had meanwhile been going forward on the distribution of fleas on Suffolk rats. Two former members of the Indian Plague Commission examined 568 rats, seventeen of which were found to be plague infected. Of 584 fleas identified, 324 were of a man-biting type, the density of fleas on rats being, in fact, very low compared with conditions during the epidemics of plague in India. A second extensive check on the rat population then took place between July and October 1911. The objective here was to define the area affected, and to this end the corpses of 15,332 rats were examined. As soon as a plague-infected rat was detected in one particular parish, no more rats were taken from that parish, this being considered sufficient evidence for the presence there of rat plague. In all, no more than thirty-five of the rats examined were diagnosed as infected, though these came from a spread of nearly thirty parishes extending from the Stour estuary to north of the River Orwell almost as far as Woodbridge.

The epizootic of rat plague in south-east Suffolk was therefore broadly extended among the local rodent population. A final check on rat fleas had established that each rat carried an average of four fleas and that about 60 per cent of these were of a man-biting species. In a general sense, and in retrospect, the danger posed to public health was, though real enough, possibly not all that acute. In his article, 'The Last

Epidemic of Plague in England? Suffolk 1906–1918', Dr David Van Zwanenberg makes the point that the

plague in rural Suffolk . . . had not behaved like the severe epidemics of the past as the authorities feared, but was like the type that exists in many remote areas of the world . . . called sylvatic or wild rodent plague. The disease is enzootic amongst the prevailing wild rodents of the area and only occasionally infects human beings. When it does infect man it tends to affect individuals or single households and . . . tends to be pneumonic rather than bubonic.

As Dr Sleigh noted in the account of the Freston outbreak which he contributed to the *British Medical Journal* of 12 November 1910:

True to description, the disease had picked out two very dirty households; and again, of all the people coming into close contact with the patients, only those who had but little respect for hygiene were infected.

Those who lived in conditions of poverty and poor housing were certainly the most vulnerable, but then, camouflaged by the picturesque tranquillity of the deep Suffolk countryside, there were many such families belonging to the agricultural community and living their lives within its depressed economy. Nevertheless, catching plague from rats or rodents in the prevailing circumstances probably depended on quite a remote mischance. That such a mischance could occur was illustrated yet again on 7 October 1911 when a sailor stationed at the naval barracks at Shotley, who had not been abroad in the past year, gutted and skinned a rabbit which he had caught on the Ipswich Road on the outskirts of Freston, and cut his finger doing so. Three days later he was in sick bay with a high temperature, a headache, and aching back and limbs. A lump in his armpit and an attack of blood-spitting preceding severe pneumonia aroused suspicions of plague and he was placed in isolation. Local Government Board officials confirmed the diagnosis, and though the sailor then survived twelve weeks of fever and abscesses among other complications, and eventually lived to be seventy-six, the disease left him virtually blind for the rest of his life.

There was one segment in the picture of plague transmission which was still not understood: the way in which a flea passed on the disease to a fresh host, animal or human. Dr Simmond had speculated that it was done through the flea defecating as it fed, but this turned out to be an insignificant cause of infection. The Oriental rat flea has a reputation for being the plague flea *par excellence*, and the final piece of the puzzle was filled in by research carried out, oddly enough, with a colony of Oriental rat fleas discovered in London in Guy's Hospital basement in 1914. The process was a complex one, but broadly it was found that a plague-infected flea suffered a blockage in its digestive system which led to its regurgitating massive doses of plague bacilli (as many as 100,000) and literally injecting these as it came to feed on a later host. A similar process is thought to occur in all species of flea implicated in the spread of plague, including the European rat flea.

The Local Government Board continued to monitor the rat population of south-east Suffolk for signs of plague up to the start of the First World War in 1914. In that year, four rats and a rabbit were found to be diseased, though these were the last rodent specimens in Suffolk to produce a positive result. A laboratory was kept open for a time, but since no further instances of rat plague came to light, it looked as though the period of alarm was over so far as *Pasteurella pestis* in Britain was concerned.

Yet the crafty bacillus still had one disagreeable trick to play, and it chose a Mrs Bugg, who lived in Warren Lane Cottages, Erwarton, only a mile or so east of Shotley, to spring it on during the last summer of the First World War. Mrs Bugg had risen as usual to do her Saturday-morning baking on 8 June 1918. Feeling chilled, she went to bed in the afternoon and rapidly developed pneumonia, from which she was dead by Thursday. Her neighbour, Mrs Garrod, who had called round to see her, fell ill on the following Sunday. Mrs Garrod's doctor was, it so happened, Dr Carey, veteran of the Freston outbreak, who detected in her symptoms of high temperature, rapid pulse and respiration and episodes of blood-spitting an unsettlingly familiar pattern. An army bacteriologist, asked to analyse a specimen of sputum, confirmed the presence of *Pasteurella pestis*, and Mrs Garrod died on the fourth day of her illness, Wednesday, 19 June.

Again, precautions were set in motion to disinfect the houses, burn bedding and clothes and place all contacts in isolation in Tattingstone Workhouse. Mrs Garrod was buried in Erwarton churchyard, where a headstone stands as her memorial half-way between the gate and the church porch. She retains the dubious distinction of being the last person in Britain to have died from naturally acquired plague as well as the last victim in Britain of the Third Pandemic which had its origins so many years before in a remote corner of Yunnan province in China.

Mankind would do well to continue to regard its old enemy with respect and wariness. The death from plague in August 1962 of a research scientist working at the Microbiological Research Establishment at Porton Down in Wiltshire hinted ominously at the use to which plague could theoretically be put in biological warfare. Widespread reservoirs of infection meanwhile remain enzootic among various species of rodent in parts of Africa and Asia, while a further legacy of the Third Pandemic was that it established the disease among prairie animals in the western United States. As a result, the occasional case of human plague still occurs among those who live or travel in the deserts of New Mexico or the foothills of the Rocky Mountains.

The fact of the matter is that the plague bacillus has, over the centuries, lost none of its vicious potential. The mechanisms or combinations of circumstance which set off the great epidemics or pandemics of the past are still only partially understood. Plague remains a shadow in the background, waiting to come into its own wherever civilized standards collapse, as happens in times of famine and war; and famine and war remain man's constant companions during the latter part of the twentieth century. It is significant that the most serious recent epidemic should have occurred in South Vietnam in 1965–70, during the Vietnam War, when there may have been as many as 175,000 cases, some of these being American servicemen.

Modern scientific medicine has produced a range of effective treatments against plague, but the question mark remains because plague can never be eradicated from the globe. As rats become increasingly resistant to poisons, fleas become increasingly resistant to insecticides and infections become increasingly resistant to antibiotics, the long-term view may hardly be seen as sanguine. *The Plague*, by Albert Camus, is one of the great metaphorical novels in twentieth-century literature, but its closing words have a disturbingly prophetic ring when its hero, Dr Rieux, feels the scepticism rise within him as he listens to the sounds of celebration from the city streets after the plague has departed:

He knew what those jubilant crowds did not know but could have learned from books: that the plague bacillus never dies or disappears for good; that it bides its time . . . and that perhaps the day would come when, for the bane and enlightening of men, it roused up its rats again and sent them forth to die in a happy city.

Chapter 8

The Paradoxes of
a Small American Disaster

On 14 February 1941, a paediatrician from Boston, Massachusetts, made a house-call in Elm Hill Park, Roxbury. Dr Stewart H. Clifford was visiting the home of a young Jewish rabbi to make a routine check on the family's three-month-old daughter, a child born prematurely who had weighed only 1·81 kilograms (4 pounds) at birth. The infant was thriving and gaining weight, and her general development looked excellent. There had been no problems, nothing noticed to cause the family concern. Yet Dr Clifford found himself examining the child with growing bewilderment and shock, glancing at the young parents as he wondered how to break the news that they had failed to notice something amiss with their baby daughter. Inexplicably, the child had become blind.

At Dr Clifford's suggestion a leading Boston ophthalmologist, Dr Paul A. Chandler, was called into consultation, and within hours the infant was admitted to the Massachusetts Eye and Ear Hospital for a more thorough examination with the baby anaesthetized. Dr Frederick Verhoeff, a leading authority on eye diseases, was also invited to be present.

As the doctors began to peer through their instruments into the baby's eyes, they could see how each one contained a thick greyish membrane covered with tiny blood-vessels.

The construction of the eye is similar to that of a box camera, a lens and refracting system at the front focusing rays of light across a small dark chamber on to a light-sensitive surface, the retina. But here the membrane seemed to be attached to the back surface of the lens, and so completely obstructed vision. The three specialists, who possessed a formidable combined weight of experience on abnormalities of the eye and diseases of infants and young children, were completely baffled. They had never seen anything remotely like it. On one point only did they feel secure in expressing an opinion: they were confident nothing could be done to restore the baby's sight.

If this tragic circumstance caused a concerned discomfiture in the ophthalmologists, it certainly prompted dismay in the paediatrician, Dr Clifford. His dismay became acute just two days after his visit to the rabbi's when he responded to an urgent request to call at the home of a prominent Boston family in Beacon Street. The cause of the crisis was a seven-month-old baby boy. During a family gathering, he was told, with relatives present from as far distant as Philadelphia, someone had remarked on how there was something odd about the baby's eyes.

Dr Clifford already knew the related case-history: the boy was the first of twins, delivered after a premature labour and weighing only 1·02 kilograms (2 pounds 4 ounces). The second-born twin, a sister, had weighed half an ounce less and died within six hours from breathing difficulties. And now, as the doctor examined the surviving infant, the assembled family awaited his verdict. There were changes in the eyes similar to those in the rabbi's daughter. For the second time within a week, Dr Clifford found himself having to tell a pair of stunned parents that their child had been struck by blindness.

In this case, another eye specialist, Dr Theodore Terry, took charge of the investigation and the child was admitted to the Children's Hospital. With Dr Chandler and Dr Verhoeff brought into consultation, the verdict confirmed Dr Clifford's suspicions. The unique character of the eye abnormality was recognized and a mystified Dr Terry could only join his colleagues in concluding that the boy's sight was permanently lost.

The two blind Boston babies did not remain isolated cases. Within a year Dr Terry had published the first clinical description of the mysterious disorder, basing his account not only on the infant boy and the rabbi's daughter, but also mentioning three other cases discovered later in the clinics of the Massachusetts Eye and Ear Hospital. The interesting factor common to them all was that each affected infant had arrived in the world prematurely, allowing Dr Terry to round off his commentary with the remark: 'In view of these findings . . . perhaps this complication should be expected in a certain percentage of premature infants. If so, some new factor has arisen in extreme prematurity to produce such a condition.'

By this stage the new disorder had acquired the resounding title of retrolental fibroplasia (or RLF for short), this seeming to be the most accurate technical description applicable to the bizarre greyish membrane formed behind the lenses of the babies' eyes. Almost inevitably, as soon as the condition was recognized, described and labelled, other victims came to be identified, enabling Dr Terry to publish by 1945 a further report on the disease based on an analysis of 117 cases, every one of which had occurred in a premature baby. Dr Terry's original conclusion appeared well justified.

The questions raised, however, were fascinating but unanswerable. Was it a new disease, or had it been occurring over many years without attracting attention? A group of retrospective studies was set in motion, though a careful re-examination of the eyes of 128 children born prematurely between 1935 and 1944 in Baltimore failed to detect a single instance. In Chicago, over 200 children born prematurely between 1922 and 1934 were visited and examined, and here just one patient with the characteristic blindness emerged, a diagnosis made sixteen years late. Similar surveys were undertaken in at least eight other American cities, as well as at Birmingham in England, and previously unrecognized examples of the condition did come to light, if only very rarely.

It even turned out to be possible to recognize the disease in historic medical literature. A scanning of medical journals published before 1940 revealed the occasional description of an inexplicable attack of blindness in a premature baby, one example having been published as early as 1820. The variety of tentative diagnoses included 'fibrous tissue cataract', 'extra-uterine endophthalmitis', 'congenital connective tissue formation in the vitreus chamber', but with the advantage of hindsight all sounded suspiciously like the now-recognized condition of retrolental fibroplasia. The conclusion was ines-capable: the disease had occurred before being discovered by Clifford, Chandler and Terry in February 1941, but luckily it had been extremely rare. Now, inexplicably, the picture was changing.

At first the medical journals contained only sporadic reports of the condition; soon, however, they were publishing a steady stream of clinical studies, case descriptions, corre-spondence, editorials, commentaries and annotations. All the original accounts came from the United States, and it seemed at first to be a disease peculiarly confined to that country. Then, in 1946, a case was diagnosed in Britain, and before long cases were also recognized in Canada and Sweden; in France, Holland, Switzerland, Spain and Italy; in South Africa, Australia and Israel. Suddenly every economically advanced country in the world was experiencing occasional instances of blindness among its smallest and frailest children. In the United States, RLF came to be regarded as one of the major problems in any premature-baby unit, at least one report speaking of an incidence as high as 12 per cent in babies weighing less than 1·40 kilograms (3 pounds).

Faced with this sudden upsurge of a new disorder, the first instinct of everyone concerned, paediatricians as well as ophthalmologists, was to see RLF as an inherent complication of prematurity, a side-effect of being born too soon. There was a strong temptation to accept as almost inevitable that a certain percentage of very immature infants were going to develop this form of blindness, and many went on to argue that the disorder had only become apparent because increasing numbers of babies of very low birth-weights were surviving to grow up and show its signs. It was rather a simplistic view, but there was much in its favour.

Retrolental fibroplasia occurred mainly in the United States, and it was certainly true that here was the country which led the world in procedures and techniques for the care of the premature baby. It was also a straightforward observation that RLF happened most often in exactly those feeble and immature infants least likely to survive without skilled or intensive neonatal care. By the 1940s, not only were more premature babies being saved, but the chances of survival for a baby of remarkably low birth-weight and extreme immaturity had increased greatly. One baby girl, born in 1936 at Palatine, Illinois, had been reared successfully despite a birth-weight as low as 340 grams (12 ounces), and in 1938 a similar success was achieved with an even lighter baby girl, born in

Britain at South Shields, and weighing only 283 grams (10 ounces).

On the other hand, several facts did not fit smoothly into this hypothesis. For one thing, not every premature baby developed RLF, while some groups of immature infants seemed completely immune. Certain premature-baby units had never seen the disorder, as at the Charity Hospital in New Orleans, where an examination of 3,000 infants failed to bring to light a single victim.

In fact, the incidence varied quite unaccountably between one group of babies and the next. It fluctuated not only from country to country, but from town to town, from hospital to hospital, even from ward to ward. There was, for instance, a high incidence in the Christian Welfare Hospital in East St Louis, Illinois, but just across the Mississippi River in St Louis, Missouri, the disease was practically unknown. It even fluctuated in time. In those hospitals where the disease occurred, the level of cases varied from year to year, even from season to season. It was quite possible for the condition to disappear from a unit altogether, only to reappear many months later. Where that happened, it seemed to reappear first in the lightest and most fragile babies, gradually spreading to the heavier infants as the incidence increased.

To deepen the mystery still further, the condition seemed to show a predilection for centres of excellence, occurring most often in the teaching hospitals of the larger universities and in more wealthy medical centres. The Cook County Hospital, in Chicago, one of the largest city hospitals in the United States, saw almost no retrolental fibroplasia, while by contrast its more richly endowed cousin, the University of Chicago Hospital, experienced an incidence of 30–40 per cent. Indeed, the association of retrolental fibroplasia with superb medical units and advanced neonatal nursing techniques was even more startling to those paediatricians who came to observe the disease from the austerity of countries still recovering from the Second World War. In their own frugally run premature units it was practically unknown, and a number of foreign physicians tentatively suggested to their hosts that here was a disease somehow connected with affluence. It was a remark both difficult to deny and impossible to explain away.

The disease seemed full of paradoxes in practically every aspect of its epidemiology. It did not run in families, but appeared to be confined predominantly to white Americans. It was present only in premature babies, yet among blacks, who suffered a far higher percentage of premature births, it was extremely uncommon. No one was yet certain when or how the disorder started. Was the premature baby born with the greyish membrane already behind the lens and obstructing vision, or did the membrane form gradually in the weeks after birth?

This latter question was tackled and answered by William and Ella Owens, a husband-and-wife team of eye specialists in the Wilmar Ophthalmological Institute of the Johns Hopkins Hospital and University at Baltimore. They made careful examinations of the eyes of more than 200 premature babies within hours of birth, none of whom showed any sign of the disorder. They then continued to monitor about half these babies, putting them through further ophthalmological examinations at monthly intervals over six months. Retrolental fibroplasia developed in only four babies, but this made it possible for the first time to study the onset and development of the disease as the Owens were able to record the formation of the characteristic accretion of membrane in each baby's eyes. The first changes were found to come about when an affected baby was, on average, two and a half months old, the earliest sign to be detected with certainty being a distortion of the small veins and arteries that supplied blood to the retina. These tiny blood vessels apparently began to swell and become twisted in their course until, within a few weeks, there was evidence of increasing damage to the actual retina, which then gradually detached itself from the eye's inner wall. As the condition progressed towards complete detachment, so the haphazard bands of fibrous tissue formed behind the lens.

At least the disease was now detectable in the early stages, before the retina became detached and destroyed. It therefore became a routine matter to check premature babies and identify those going blind. Yet the statistics as they emerged proved astounding; the incidence was evidently increasing month by month, while a few premature-baby units found as many as 70 per cent of infants showing early signs. Back in 1943, Dr Terry had suggested that RLF could be caused by too early an exposure of the immature eye to light. Now a disconcerting question arose: might the brightly illuminated instruments of the ophthalmologists be triggering off the disease?

With the infants at risk now known, hope was raised of finding a form of treatment, but since no general agreement about the cause existed, there was nothing on which to base a rational therapy. Attempts at prevention or cure needed to be empirical, founded entirely on the unproven convictions and guesses of the individual doctor in charge. And as so often happens with diseases for which no really effective cure exists, a multiplicity of treatments was put forward. It was felt, for example, that the eyes of premature infants might suffer from lack of oxygen. The best treatment would therefore be to nurse the baby in the oxygen-enriched atmosphere of an incubator: and, indeed, at least one highly respected pathologist, after studying the eye damage, stated that it looked like a consequence of oxygen deficiency. Others suggested that it was the sudden removal of a baby from intensive oxygen treatment which was responsible and recommended a more gradual reduction in oxygen concentrations. At the Johns Hopkins Hospital, the Owens became convinced that a form of vitamin E (alphatocopherol) would arrest the disease, while in New York, a newly discovered hormone (adrenocorticotrophic or ACTH) came into favour. ACTH, it was reported, showed signs of inhibiting the inflammatory processes of the body and so diminishing scar-tissue formation.

Yet the results yielded by these varied treatments were conflicting and confusing, almost every suggestion apparently producing a harvest of successful cures, followed all too quickly by a crop of frustrating failures. With certain infants, paediatricians found themselves watching wonderingly as every sign of the disorder gradually receded and disappeared. With others, they stood by helplessly as their favoured method entirely failed to halt the destructive progression of changes in a baby's eyes.

An explanation for these baffling results came at last from the Wilmar Institute of Ophthalmology at the Johns Hopkins Hospital in Baltimore, the husband-and-wife team of the Owens once again providing the answer. Through repeated serial studies, William Owens discovered that, with many premature infants, the early changes of RLF did not invariably progress to retinal detachment and blindness. In many babies, in fact in a vast majority, every sign disappeared spontaneously. Eventually it was accepted that nearly 85 per cent of babies with early changes recovered without treatment, leaving only 15 per cent to progress to unavoidable blindness.

It now became hard to believe in any of the treatments so

far advocated. One of them was even shown to be positively harmful when a cautiously conducted trial of ACTH in New York demonstrated that while failing to help RLF, it also positively diminished a premature baby's chances of survival.

By now the outbreak had reached an epidemic scale. During 1950, in New York State alone, 110 babies were registered blind, while throughout the world as many as 2,500 babies were blinded annually. Simple calculations suggested that about a further 15,000 babies who suffered from early signs fortunately recovered, but the fact remained that, in less than a decade, RLF had changed from being among the rarest diseases to the commonest cause of blindness in childhood. In the United States, various administrative departments were already starting to make discreet projections and long-term plans to provide the increased facilities needed to care for a growing population of the permanently blind.

For doctors in charge of neonatal units, the disease had turned into a nightmare, heralding growing feelings of disquiet, self-doubt and helplessness. One spectre above all was raising its disturbing head: that RLF could be among those conditions called iatrogenic, meaning a disorder caused by medical treatment intended to help the patient.

The paradoxes were deepening, for few environments could have been more protective than that surrounding a premature infant in an incubator. Every facet of it was monitored and regulated, and nothing happened which was not the result of a carefully calculated decision, from the temperature and humidity of the air breathed to the composition of milk fed, from the posture in which a child was nursed to the selection of drugs administered. And yet it was precisely these 'privileged' little patients, nursed in such ideal circumstances, who were most at hazard.

It was a fact that the finest neonatal units in the world held a high percentage of babies destined to go blind, while in hospitals with only limited facilities, and even in humble homes like that in Ontario where the Dionne quintuplets had been reared in laundry baskets behind the stove, retrolental fibroplasia was absent. The conclusion was inescapable. Somewhere around 1940 the painstakingly evolved high-technology techniques of modern intensive care for the premature baby had taken a wrong turning.

The French critic and scholar Adrien Baillet recounts in his book *Judgements of Scholars Concerning the Principal Works of Authors* (Paris, 1722) a story from the eleventh century of the Roman Republic

of Fortunio Liceri, whose mother gave birth to him long before the ordinary time during the fatigue and shocks of a sea voyage. This foetus was no larger than the palm of your hand, but his father who was a physician, having examined it, had carried it to the place which was to be the end of his voyage. There he had other physicians see it. They found that there was lacking nothing essential to life, and his father undertook to finish Nature's task and to work at the formation of the child with the same skill that men exhibited in hatching chickens in Egypt. He instructed the nurse in all that she had to do in the maintaining of exactly measured artificial heat and the requirements for his general care and feeding. He [the child] lived to be seventy-nine years of age and distinguished himself in science by a large number of works.

There have always been premature babies, and they have always caused problems. Even Hippocrates, writing in the fourth century BC, was driven to observe gloomily and dogmatically how 'no foetus coming into the world before the seventh month of pregnancy can be saved'. Today it is considered more accurate to assess the maturity of a baby by its birth-weight, rather than by what is often an imprecise estimate of the duration of a pregnancy. A premature baby has been defined as an infant weighing less than 2·5 kilograms (5½ pounds) at birth, though this figure could need adjusting slightly for some populations and racial groups where the average birth-weight differs from that general in the more economically advanced nations.

The care of such tiny infants inevitably presents many delicate problems. They are sensitive to the slightest changes in environment; they may well be incapable of maintaining a stable independent body temperature. Smaller babies may be unable to suck, or even to swallow, and therefore can only be nourished by tube-feeding. An immature baby may not even have developed a cough-reflex, creating the danger of secretions or regurgitated feed being inhaled into its lungs. Premature infants are particularly prone to breathing diffi- culties, which may include episodes of irregular respiration or even frightening attacks when breathing is temporarily arrested and the baby turns blue (cyanosis). The immaturity of internal organs like the liver leaves the baby vulnerable to such metabolic and biochemical dangers as low blood sugar or severe jaundice. Any premature baby is extremely suscep- tible to infections that may be hard to detect yet which need prompt, effective treatment, while the most tried and tested of drugs can present unexpected hazards when given to an embryonic charge.

The intensive care of these miniature patients has to be a gentle and delicate craft, and it was inevitable that the resuscitation of a human being smaller in size than the average doll should have called into existence its own branch of medical specialization. Despite an ancient and classical history, and attempts during the Middle Ages to nurse immature infants wrapped in lamb's wool or immersed in jars of feathers, the care of premature babies was still in 1940 a young science finding its way. Practically all the techniques of modern neonatology had evolved over a period of less than seventy years, and only the administration of oxygen had a longer history. Oxygen was discovered and named during the 1770s, and by 1780 a French doctor, Chaussier, was experimenting with the gas on new-born infants who failed to establish normal breathing.

Interestingly enough, most early advances in the care of prematurity were made in France. In 1857, a tub-like metal cot with double walls heated by warm water was designed in Bordeaux for nursing the frailer new-born. By 1880 the cot, with its water-jacket, had been replaced by an incubator, a large wooden cabinet capable of holding several babies at once. This had a compartment heated by warm air, while a window in the top made it possible to peep at the faces of babies inside. The idea was adapted from a warming chamber used to rear poultry, the actual cabinet being constructed by the director of the Paris Zoo. In 1884, Tarnier, the Parisian obstetrician who pioneered the incubator, introduced the technique of tube-feeding. Thus, for the first time, attempts were made to save even the feeblest infants by feeding human milk directly into their stomachs.

The first unit in the world to be devoted exclusively to the care of the premature baby, a so-called nursery for 'weaklings', was founded in 1893 at the Hôpital Maternité in Paris, a second centre being opened at the Clinique Tarnier within five years. An epidemic of respiratory infection at the Hôpital Maternité in 1896 led to the introduction of such procedures as the isolation of sick babies, the wearing of special overalls by attendants and the precaution of preparing all feeds in a separate 'sterilizing room'.

By the 1890s, the spectacle of small swaddled infants being

nursed in rows of incubators by specially garbed attendants was considered so novel that exhibitions were organized in several leading provincial cities of France. Elsewhere in Europe, in 1896, premature babies were borrowed from the Charity Hospital in Berlin to be nursed in incubators as an attraction at the World Exposition in the city, while, in 1897, a similar display was organized at Earl's Court, London, for the Victorian Era Exhibition. With the new century, this curious medical side-show reached America. In Buffalo, New York, an imposing building was built to house an incubator exhibition with live premature infants as part of the Pan-American Exhibition of 1901. The exhibition later became a regular feature at Coney Island every summer, visitors being charged an admission fee of 25 cents.

The earliest permanent centre for the care of immature infants in the United States was opened in 1922 in Chicago. This was the Sarah Morris Premature Baby Unit, which, during the first five years of its existence, was able to save only half the small patients admitted to its care. By the mid 1930s, however, the unit was recording a survival rate of practically 80 per cent.

By the 1930s, premature-baby units had become virtually sacred ground, reserved to the initiates of their mysteries. The premature baby was now nursed almost entirely hidden inside an envelope of soft woollen clothes and isolated from the outside world by the glass walls of a cubicle. It was handled and disturbed as seldom as possible, touched only by a hierarchy of dedicated, experienced nurses, whose humanity was thoroughly camouflaged by hygienic masks and gowns.

The trouble with these highly protective surroundings was that they presented an obstacle not only to observing the baby's condition but also to studying its diseases. Then, however, during the 1940s, a new generation of incubators came into use. These were literally designed to encapsulate each infant within an individually regulated atmosphere. The baby now lay inside a transparent compartment in which it could even be tended and fed without the incubator needing to be opened.

With the advent of this new protective capsule, the multiple layers of clothing came to be recognized as an unnecessary impediment to nursing and so were quietly discarded. All at once the premature baby became visible. Overnight, nurses and physicians discovered the almost mesmeric quality radiated by the spectacle of a tiny human being struggling to live. Every hesitant breath could be observed, every twitch or movement of the limbs noted, every change in skin colour or muscle tone detected and analysed. Total observation was for the first time possible.

By now the regular care of a premature baby might include such treatments as the careful use of a high-protein diet, the administration of iron and desperately needed vitamins, or an occasional transfusion of minute amounts of blood or plasma. In some centres hormones were used, while in others penicillin was injected almost as a matter of routine to protect babies against 'infection'.

It was a complex business, involving fine balances of judgement, but with each year that passed it became progressively more likely that a premature baby would survive. In the overall context of these achievements, the fact that so many tiny patients were going blind was intensely distressing.

A casual visitor to the premature unit in the Babies Hospital, New York, in 1951, would have been intrigued to see how each baby was provided with an eye-patch. Nine years earlier it had been suggested that too early an exposure of the immature eye to light could be the cause of retrolental fibroplasia, and at last the matter was being put to the test. Twenty-two premature infants were each equipped with an eye-patch, placed over one eye within hours of birth and remaining in position until the baby's discharge from the unit several weeks later. Nevertheless a proportion of these babies continued to develop retrolental fibroplasia, the disease occurring just as severely in the protected as in the unprotected eye. A second experiment, with thirty-five babies who had both eyes covered, similarly failed to prevent cases of retrolental fibroplasia from occurring. Exposure to light clearly played no role.

This somewhat negative piece of information was at least unequivocal, and four other studies meanwhile reached a similar conclusion. In other areas, however, there was a degree of chaos over contradicting results. Many parallel studies, which seemed at first to yield useful observations and significant leads for further research, gave entirely different results when repeated. Over and over again the results of time-consuming trials were flatly denied by findings from precisely similar trials conducted elsewhere.

By this stage a world-wide debate was taking place in the pages of the medical journals. Each phase of a premature baby's existence was being scrutinized, from the moment of conception to the period two or three months after birth when retrolental fibroplasia became apparent. The ages and economic standing of parents were considered, as were the seasons and months of conception, the use of drugs and X-rays in pregnancy, the occurrence of maternal illness or obstetric abnormality, the type of anaesthetic used in the delivery room, methods of resuscitation and the various illnesses and treatments which an infant could experience. At least fifty or sixty possible causes put forward were vigorously investigated.

The first tentative glimpse of the truth came, somewhat unexpectedly, from one of those foreign observers who originally linked retrolental fibroplasia with affluence. Among them was Victoria Mary Crosse, a redoubtable doctor who organized the United Kingdom's first premature-baby unit at Sorrento Hospital, Birmingham, in 1931, and who later fascinatedly noted how RLF only became common in England after the inception of the National Health Service in 1948. It seemed a remarkable coincidence that the epidemic should have arrived at precisely the moment when government subsidies made it possible to introduce expensive technological innovations into the premature-baby nursery. Dr Crosse pondered on the matter and arrived at a shrewd suspicion. In due course her musings reached the ears of an Australian paediatrician, Dr Kate Campbell, who held a special responsibility for the care of new-born infants in Melbourne's hospitals.

One of these, the Women's Hospital, possessed a newly built nursery where oxygen was piped into the ward. It was further equipped with efficient 'oxygen-cots' in which concentrations of 40–60 per cent of oxygen could be achieved with ease. For several years doctors had known how a small infant can become quite short of oxygen without necessarily showing the most obvious symptoms of oxygen deficiency, such as a blueish tinge in the complexion or distressed breathing. As a result, it became usual for oxygen to be administered in any case where there was concern about a baby's condition. Yet, at the Women's Hospital in Melbourne, practice had taken the process one step further. It was a matter of course for nursing staff there to give oxygen liberally to all immature babies, even without any immediately demanding circumstance.

By contrast, in the other hospital under Dr Campbell's care, premature babies were nursed in electrically heated cots and oxygen was only given when needed by a small rubber funnel or by a catheter placed inside the baby's nose; or even, on occasion, by an improvised oxygen-tent. It was impossible by such means to reach any high concentration of the gas, and furthermore it was usual in the second hospital for the finance department to charge patients for oxygen supplied. Not surprisingly, far less oxygen was used in this unit than in its equivalent at the Women's Hospital.

When Dr Campbell seized on the chance to compare incidences of RLF in the two nurseries, she turned up some startling implications. In the Women's Hospital, 19 per cent of immature infants developed retrolental fibroplasia; in the other hospital, only 7 per cent suffered eye damage. The results could not stand as an experiment or a trial, but only as a retrospective survey, for groups of babies nursed in different hospitals were being compared, and the incidence of retrolental fibroplasia was notoriously erratic in its variations from hospital to hospital. When Dr Campbell published an article on her findings in the *Medical Journal of Australia* of 14 July 1951 – an article which fully acknowledged the original inspiration of Dr Crosse – she was proving nothing concerning the culpability of oxygen, but she was providing some very interesting signposts.

In the meantime, in Washington, DC, a clinical trial was being set up at the Gallagher Municipal Hospital to find out whether the number of cases could be reduced by limiting oxygen use. It was planned not as a simple survey of past experience, like that undertaken by Kate Campbell, but as a rigorously controlled experiment. All premature babies admitted to the nursery were to be allocated to one of two groups. In the first, oxygen would be given freely, concentrations as high as 65–70 per cent being maintained in the incubator for as long as four to seven weeks. The second group, on the other hand, was to be nursed in incubation where oxygen concentration never exceeded 40 per cent, the gas being used for as short a time as the infant's condition allowed. In everything else, treatment of the two groups would be identical.

Almost at once the project ran into criticism and obstruction, one research foundation declaring itself unwilling to finance a trial which, it felt, would place in jeopardy the lives of those babies who were to be given only a curtailed supply. These fears were shared by many nurses at the hospital, and the experiment was sometimes even sabotaged by staff turning on oxygen supplies to all the incubators at night as soon as their activities were unsupervised.

Despite these set-backs and interferences, the trial, originally designed to run for three years, was by the end of the first year producing results so striking that the figures were published at once. While 7 per cent of babies nursed in high concentrations of oxygen had gone blind, none of those nursed with minimal oxygen suffered a trace of eye damage.

Publication of the results caused widespread consternation. These findings needed to be confirmed or disproved with minimum delay, for all over the United States babies were, at that moment, being nursed in high concentrations of oxygen.

The 1952 annual meeting of the American Academy of Ophthalmology and Otolaryngology brought the subject forward for urgent debate, most of those present agreeing that a large-scale experimental trial was an urgent necessity. Early in 1953, a majority of American paediatricians and ophthalmologists involved in the study of retrolental fibroplasia therefore gathered at Bethesda, Maryland, under the auspices of the National Institute of Neurological Diseases and Blindness. Opinion was still divided, some doctors feeling that the matter was settled beyond doubt by the Gallagher Municipal Hospital trial, while others, like the Gallagher nurses before them, feared it would be extremely unsafe to reduce doses of oxygen. A majority, however, came out in favour of a comprehensive scientific trial, conducted on a national scale.

The National Cooperative Study, as it came to be known, was set in motion on 1 July 1953. The sample of eighteen hospitals selected stretched across the United States from the Boston Lying-In Hospital in the north to the New Orleans Charity Hospital in the south, the study being controlled from a co-ordination centre in the Kresege Eye Institute, Detroit. It ran for exactly a year, finishing on 30 June 1954, during which period 1,420 babies weighing less than 1·5 kilograms (3 pounds 5 ounces) were born in or admitted to the wards of the eighteen sample hospitals, 786 of these infants surviving the first forty-eight hours of life. This large population of tiny babies was to make a basis for the experiment, and it was decided that, for every baby nursed with routine levels of oxygen, two others were to be submitted to a regime in which the administration of supplemental oxygen was drastically reduced. The trial was designed so that any sign of an increased safety risk could be quickly detected.

The results could only be assessed statistically out of the coded information deposited at the co-ordinating centre in Detroit, and hence these were awaited with much impatience. It took almost another three months before the findings could be presented, and on 19 September 1954 they were finally laid before the fifty-ninth annual meeting of the American Academy of Ophthalmology and Otolaryngology in New York City. They were dramatic and indisputable: high

concentrations of oxygen greatly increased the risk of immature babies going blind. A premature infant was, in fact, three
times more likely to develop RLF if nursed with what had
come to be regarded as a standard administration of oxygen.

Several related facts were also established. To begin with,
it was not the concentration of oxygen which mattered, but
the length of time over which it was given. For practical
purposes there seemed to be no safe concentration of oxygen.
Wherever supplemental oxygen was prescribed, the risk
increased of retrolental fibroplasia developing. The risk itself
became greater, however, with the number of days over
which the gas was administered. It was also shown how the
rate of withdrawing oxygen was totally unimportant. Finally,
twins were shown to be particularly at risk, displaying
an exceptional vulnerability to the disease.

Over time it came to be understood how oxygen could
precipitate blindness. With high concentrations, damage was
caused to the cells lining the smaller blood vessels, the
capillaries and tiny arteries at the back of the immature eye.
The lining cells gradually swelled until the minute blood
vessels became obstructed or even obliterated. Now the retina
and tissues at the back of the eye were starved of blood and
oxygen, and it was in an attempt to overcome the disturbances
in the circulation of the blood that there came about, in those
cases which progressed to blindness, an active but disorderly
overgrowth of new blood vessels. Haemorrhages and the
exudation of fluid then occurred, stripping the retina from its
attachment.

In short, the ultimate paradox had been reached: it was the
administration of a high concentration of oxygen which could
cause sensitive tissues at the back of the eye to become
oxygen starved and so lead to tragic results.

The reverberations from the National Cooperative Study

were immediate, the turn-about in medical practice spectacular. Oxygen all at once came to be treated with uneasy respect and caution in every premature-baby unit in the world. Its administration was strictly monitored and curtailed, and only those babies suffering from obvious respiratory or cardiac distress were allowed supplemental oxygen, and then no more than in the lowest concentration and for the shortest period needed to relieve symptoms.

The impact on RLF was equally dramatic. Month by month the incidence plummeted. About 300,000 babies a year were born in New York State, and, of those born in 1952, 168 lost their sight, the equivalent figure for 1953 being 167. Yet for those born in 1955, the first full year after the study, only three babies were subsequently registered as blind. This almost magical disappearance of the disease showed the same pattern in every town, city and state. By the late 1950s it was possible to downgrade RLF to an uncommon if not exactly rare disease, and in various state departments blueprints for expanding amenities for blind children and adults were quietly shelved with relief. As Stewart Duke-Elder triumphantly observed in the tenth volume of his monumental work on diseases of the eye, 'never in the history of ophthalmology has a blinding condition become so quickly widespread and equally rapidly been abolished'.

The problem of retrolental fibroplasia, it seemed, was solved. Yet, by the early 1960s, it began to grow equally certain that the story was by no means over and done with. Accumulating stacks of reports suggested that the fears of the rebel night staff at the Gallagher Municipal Hospital could have been well founded, their obstruction of the research foundation a far-sighted storm-warning.

Early trials failed to detect any increased risk to the premature baby from curtailing oxygen supply, yet events appeared to be vindicating the reservations of the more hesitant group of physicians at Bethesda. Precise statistics revealed that, even as the incidence of retrolental fibroplasia fell, so had morbidity and mortality risen among premature infants. With oxygen supplies restricted and retrolental fibroplasia becoming an infrequent disease, increasing numbers of premature babies were either showing signs of brain damage from anoxia or dying from respiratory distress. By 1973, after a careful survey and some computation, Victoria Mary Crosse felt driven to make the simple and stark statement that 'it would seem that each sighted baby may have cost some sixteen deaths'. Coming from a dedicated, gifted paediatrician, it sounded like a cry of bitter self-reproach.

Doctors now found themselves facing a stark dilemma. In caring for the smallest premature babies, they were being forced to shepherd their frail charges along a narrow path of uncertain hazard, avoiding the pit of blindness on the one side and the abyss of brain damage and death on the other. If any secure middle way was to be discovered, both the upper and lower limits of safety in oxygen therapy needed to be defined precisely.

The epidemic had been abolished simply by curtailing supplies of oxygen. In fact, in the clinical circumstances of the 1950s, it had turned out to be extremely difficult to come by accurate, repeated measurements of the actual concentration of oxygen within an incubator. By the late 1960s, the technology of the premature-baby unit had advanced. Modern instruments and microtechniques now made it possible not only to monitor with close accuracy the concentration of oxygen inside the incubator, but even to study the partial pressure of oxygen within the babies' arterial blood. Physicians could thus measure precisely the amount of oxygen being carried by the bloodstream to the eyes and brain of their tiny patients. Armed with this clinical tool, it seemed reasonable to suppose that it should become possible for them to administer exactly the right amount of oxygen. All that was necessary to give this information was one further ambitious, carefully organized trial to chart the limits of oxygen saturation which should be maintained in babies' arterial blood.

The second National Cooperative Study began in 1969. It ran for three years, involving twenty-seven investigators working at five university centres and having 719 premature infants under their observation. The trial was intended to define two simple measurements: first, the lowest level of oxygen saturation in a baby's arterial blood capable of provoking RLF, and second, the shortest period of exposure to this oxygen level likely to cause the disease. The upper margins of safe oxygen administration to immature infants would thus, it was hoped, be established.

This time the trial proved a sad disappointment. Its findings, after the results were evaluated and its report prepared by a team of ten writers, took five years to reach publication. It entirely failed to discover any correlation between arterial-blood oxygen levels and the onset of RLF. No significant difference could be discovered between the oxygen concentration in the blood of the infants who went blind and that in those whose eyes remained normal. While RLF occurred, as anticipated, more often where there were high concentrations and prolonged administration of oxygen, occasional onsets appeared in babies nursed only briefly in quite low concentrations.

In fact, the trial confirmed the findings of the first study: that there was no such thing as a safe concentration, no 'cutoff' point below which RLF could be relied on not to occur.

Indeed, as the early unrecognized cases described in the pages of nineteenth-century medical journals already indicated, there were even occasions when retrolental fibroplasia happened in premature babies never exposed to oxygen treatment. In clinics scattered across the world, rare but authentic examples were now being discovered of premature babies developing the disease after being nursed in nothing more concentrated than atmospheric air.

The physicians remained firmly on the horns of their dilemma: there was no such thing as a safe middle ground in oxygen therapy. Where there was reason for concern about the welfare of a premature infant, paediatricians could only choose between desperate options. They could withhold oxygen treatment for as long as they dared, risking injury to the brain or even death for their patients, or they could administer the gas, gambling on the chance of the child escaping without eye damage. It remained a purely 'clinical' decision, a matter for personal judgement, with inevitable burdens of responsibility, doubt and even guilt.

To complicate matters further, new photographic and X-ray techniques revealed the startling fact that the early reversible blood-vessel changes associated with the disease occurred far more often in premature babies than had been realized. One investigator in Denver, Colorado, using the new techniques to study the eyes of fifty-two teenagers born prematurely both during and after the epidemic, found only three individuals with completely normal eyes. It was clear that the early vascular changes were an extremely common abnormality in premature babies, whether or not they had been treated with oxygen.

The problem of retrolental fibroplasia could at last be seen whole – and it moved from paradox to enigma. How was it, then, that every premature baby did not go blind? Why, in so many immature infants, did the early vascular changes subside without proceeding to retinal detachment and fibrosis, and ultimately to blindness?

This, as Sherlock Holmes would no doubt have pointed out, was another of those cases of 'the dog that did not bark in the night'. The initial vascular changes certainly occurred in the eyes of most premature babies. In some instances, particularly among the lightest and most immature infants and those who had been exposed to oxygen, the microscopic changes could become the starting-point for a progressive disease which ultimately destroyed the eye. In a vast majority of cases, however, before any serious damage was done, the disease process was mysteriously arrested or even reversed. Indeed, most infants who had developed the vascular changes of the disease, even those exposed to high concentrations of oxygen for prolonged periods during the retrolental fibroplasia epidemic, suffered no retinal scarring or loss of vision.

There had to be some other factor besides extreme immaturity and oxygen administration which governed the outcome of the disease process in each patient. There had to be something which protected most premature babies from the full ravages. Once this factor could be identified and controlled, the conundrum presented would be fully resolved. Yet to this day that factor remains an unknown quantity.

The story of retrolental fibroplasia presents us with a scientific morality, but like all the best parables it contains no clear-cut distinction between right and wrong. It tells of how a confident technological advance took several steps in front of any understanding of its full consequences. The dilemma it created still stands and places paediatricians in the troubling circumstances of having to take calculated risks with the destinies of the most touchingly vulnerable of their patients. But while retrolental fibroplasia remains imperfectly understood, it has at least now been safely returned to the category of a very rare disease. The fundamental tragedy is that it took forty years and over 10,000 blind individuals simply to understand the nature of the questions which it posed.

Chapter 9

The Beetle of Aphrodite

During the late evening of Monday, 26 May 1954, a 27-year-old typist was admitted to St James's Hospital, Balham, in south London. She was considerably distressed and was clearly desperately ill. There was a suspicion of poisoning.

This unmarried, rather shy and self-conscious young woman lived a well-regulated life with her parents in Wimbledon, about three miles from the hospital. Each morning she would catch a No. 93 bus into central London, where she worked as a secretary and typist for a wholesale chemists in the Euston Road. She had been with the firm since leaving school at thirteen, and now worked with twenty-two other women and four men under the direction of an office manager in the company's large main office.

Her day, that Monday, had gone as usual until, at about 2.30 in the afternoon, shortly after the staff got back from lunch, the office manager generously produced a bag of cubes of coconut-icing and offered pieces round to several of the girls. The office manager, a busy rather self-important man of forty-four, worked in the main office itself, sharing a standard bench type of desk with several secretaries and typists. His place was singled out only by the fact of it being next to the wall and that he sat on a wooden, swivel office chair with arms rather than on one of the standard adjustable-backed metal stools of the typists.

About ten minutes after the coconut-icing had been handed round, one of the younger girls began to feel ill, complaining of pains in her abdomen and of nausea. She was normally a cheerful nineteen-year-old, only recently recruited, who had already achieved some distinction by winning a beauty queen contest while on holiday in Margate. The fact that she was engaged to be married also made her a centre of office attention. By three o'clock she was vomiting and needed to be taken to the first-aid room, escorted by the 27-year-old typist from Wimbledon, herself beginning to feel unwell. The younger girl was given a teaspoon of bicarbonate of soda stirred into a glass of water, but complained at once that it only made her pains worse. She was now suffering an intolerable burning sensation in her mouth and throat. Blisters began to form round her mouth, speech became difficult, swallowing impossible. The typist escorting her was also starting to experience some more acute symptoms including violent spasms of abdominal cramp and waves of nausea followed by bouts of vomiting. Her mouth and throat felt as if they were starting to burn.

Back in the main office there was a scene of growing consternation as the office manager slumped at his desk. After he had complained of headache, his face had grown mottled, peculiar blisters had come up on his cheek and lips and he now appeared unconscious. An ambulance was summoned to drive him to University College Hospital, whither the nineteen-year-old typist, also growing steadily worse, was likewise taken. The older girl, however, managed to rally as her symptoms subsided a little. She was anxious only to get home, she said, and at her request a taxi was called. In the taxi the pain and nausea returned and she was soon overcome by spasms of stomach cramps and retching. Despite all efforts to restrain herself, she found herself vomiting again and again, and when she reached home at about six o'clock she needed to be carried up the stairs to the family's second-floor flat. A watching neighbour was startled by the contrast between the grey pallor of her face and the bright red of her coat and beret.

By now she was vomiting blood. At 7.30 her doctor arrived, a woman general practitioner who was shocked by the condition in which she found her patient. On her advice the typist at last allowed herself to be transferred to hospital, and at 9.30 that evening, seven hours after symptoms began, she arrived in St James's Casualty Department in a serious state of shock: pale, collapsed, and with a weak rapid pulse and low blood pressure. An injection of morphine was given and a gentle attempt made to wash out her stomach, after which there seemed to be a slight improvement and it became possible to move her into one of the wards. Yet, within minutes, she was vomiting about half a pint of fresh blood as her condition again deteriorated.

Five miles away, doctors were battling with an almost identical problem at University College Hospital, where the nineteen-year-old had arrived at five o'clock, in violent pain and bringing up bloodstained mucus. She also had a diarrhoea. One corner of her mouth showed a curious blistering of the skin, and when the mouth was opened her tongue was found to be grossly inflamed and swollen. The most startling symptom, however, was that the lining of her tongue had grown white and was peeling away, as was the lining of throat and palate. It was impossible to see down the throat because of the damage done to its walls and the accumulation of bloodstained mucus. Her windpipe was painful and acutely tender, and it was impossible even to think of passing down a stomach-tube to wash out the stomach, so swollen, weeping and inflamed were the throat and passageways. She was given an injection of morphine and put on an infusion of intravenous fluids.

By late evening, the medical teams at the respective hospitals were growing aware of their shared problems. Each one faced a mystifying clinical picture of a young woman suffering the most brutal form of chemical injury: severe corrosive poisoning. It was obvious both had swallowed something so irritant that it was burning and destroying the linings of all the passageways from mouth and throat down to the stomach.

Acute corrosive poisoning is a highly uncommon though well-recognized medical emergency. Few people make the mistake of swallowing something so caustic or acid that it burns the lips and mouth on contact, and it is rare even as an instrument of attempted suicide, occurring only in the most mentally or emotionally disturbed. Yet here, in the offices of a firm specializing in the manufacture and distribution of chemicals, three apparently inexplicable examples of exactly this type of poisoning had erupted simultaneously.

The police, already informed, were by 9.16 that evening questioning the office manager. He was extremely distressed, but appeared to be in a less serious state than the girls. His face was mottled, and he had blisters on his face and cheek close to the mouth, but he luckily seemed to be escaping any internal effects. There had been no damage to the mucous membrane of his mouth or tongue, no abdominal pain or vomiting. Although close to incoherence, he was the only one of the victims still capable of speech.

It was upon the coconut-icing that initial police suspicions fell, reinforced by a remark made by the office manager himself: 'It must have been the coconut-icing.' He then made a statement to the investigating officer, Detective Superintendent John Jamieson, describing how he bought the coconut-icing before returning to the office and sharing it out among his staff. In the office itself, the police had meanwhile recovered the paper bag in which the sweets were carried, and found it even contained two uneaten pieces. Under the gaze of an assistant manager, hastily summoned from home, they subjected the desks of typists and office manager to a minute investigation, brushing the fine debris and tiny fallen flakes of coconut-icing from the surfaces into small, carefully labelled envelopes. Checking the manager's drawer, they found a pair of scissors with what looked like a smear of coconut-icing across the blades. In the first-aid room, they took possession of the bottle from which bicarbonate of soda had been dispensed. At the sweet shop in nearby Hampstead Road, they confiscated the entire stock of chocolate-covered pink and white coconut-icing. Seven pounds of that particular batch had already been sold.

By this time it was clear that several other girls from the main office had eaten pieces of coconut-icing without ill-effect. Nor were any complaints emerging from among other of the sweet shop's customers. In any case, forensic tests on the two uneaten pieces proved entirely negative. Neither the bicarbonate of soda from the first-aid room nor these pieces of coconut-icing were contaminated by any harmful substance. It seemed for the moment that speculation on the nature of the poison must remain in the hands of the doctors fighting to aid the victims.

At University College Hospital, the attention of Professor Charles Rimmington had already been caught by a fascinating observation. The pain caused by swallowing an acid or caustic chemical should, in the ordinary way, begin almost at once, any damage to the mucous membranes of throat and oesophagus happening practically instantaneously. The cases of these two young women, however, had shown a time-lag of several minutes, even a quarter of an hour, before discomfort began. Visible signs of injury to mouth-lining membranes had become manifest even more slowly.

It was the observation of delayed symptoms which sparked off a startling but inspired guess in Professor Rimmington's mind. There was one extremely rare form of corrosive poisoning in which the onset of symptoms was delayed; only twenty-four cases had been reported in the present century. Its clinical picture was usually complicated within a few hours by symptoms of kidney damage, such as the passage of bloodstained urine or even a complete suppression of urine formation. Should renal symptoms such as these develop in either girl, then, he knew, his guess would be correct and they would be dealing with a classical case.

It was a classical case in more senses than one. It had, indeed, a famous and remarkable precedent which began on Tuesday, 30 June 1772, when Jean-Pierre Chomel, *Lieutenant Général criminel* at the Seneschal's Court in Marseille, received a written order to investigate an allegation of poisoning.

The victim was a 25-year-old prostitute, Marguerite Coste, who lived in the rue Saint-Ferreol le Vieux. Chomel found the girl incapable of moving from her bed and distressed by repeated bouts of vomiting. Her bed-linen was soiled by the blackish congealed matter which she was bringing up. She had already been ill for three days.

The story which she told Chomel was as disturbing as it was intriguing. On Saturday, 27 June, at about nine o'clock in the evening, she had been visited by a nobleman accompanied by his manservant. The nobleman she judged to be in his early thirties, a blond man of medium height who wore a grey dress-coat and eye-catching silken breeches the colour of marigolds. He had a dress-sword and carried a gold-headed cane, while his valet, a tall pock-marked man, was dressed in a yellow and blue striped sailor suit.

The nobleman made himself comfortable, depositing his cane and removing his sword before sitting at the foot of the bed with Marguerite Coste on a chair next to him. During the lengthy conversation which followed, the nobleman offered her some sweets from a small gold-rimmed cannister. These she later described as 'tablets, rather like sweet aniseed balls'. She took a few and ate them. When offered more she at first declined, but eventually let herself be persuaded into eating all those remaining. Soon afterwards the nobleman asked whether she was aware of feeling anything in her stomach or chest. Then, abruptly, he proposed that he should 'take possession of her from behind and in many other even more horrible ways'. Marguerite Coste claimed that she refused, but admitted that she eventually allowed him to have intercourse and 'amuse himself with her body', even though his manservant remained in the room. Nobleman and man-servant then withdrew, leaving six francs on the table.

Hardly had they left the room before Marguerite felt as if her stomach was on fire. Within minutes she was vomiting copiously, bringing up 'substances of different colours and most often blackish substances' which had an acrid taste and stank abominably. (This unpleasant black material was undoubtedly altered blood partially digested by the stomach acid.) Her vomiting continued through that Saturday night, and early on Sunday morning she summoned the widow who owned the house and who was her landlady. The woman noticed how the bedcover was flooded with blackish vomit and found that, although Marguerite Coste asked for some tea, she could not retain even warm water in her stomach. By evening, when the doctor was called, she was suffering severe pains in stomach and abdomen.

In response to her pleas for relief, the doctor administered sweet almond oil, but the vomiting continued without mercy. By Tuesday she was still vomiting, and her condition had grown so pitiable that her landlady, fearing she might die, informed the authorities. That evening Marguerite Coste again vomited several times while being questioned and making her statement, and Chomel was able to inspect the copious, black, fetid material she produced, carefully collecting a sample in a bottle and sealing it with the seal of the Seneschal's Court.

The next day, Wednesday, 1 July, she was visited by a physician and a surgeon appointed to examine her. They found her 'laid on her back in her bed, her eyes glistening, her face red and burning, her tongue moist and coated by a whitish mucus, her pulse hard and frequent'. She was complaining of an excruciating pain and tenderness in the region of the stomach, while beside the bed was a basin full of blackish vomit. The doctors therefore prescribed what they considered to be soothing, mucilaginous liquids, to be administered both as medicines and as enemas.

In the meantime, the *Lieutenant Général criminel* was making further inquiries at a house of ill-repute in the rue d'Aubagne on the corner with the rue des Capucins. Here Chomel had stumbled over what seemed to be a separate yet related happening. In his questioning of four young prostitutes he was garnering details of an extraordinary sequence of events which had occurred earlier on Saturday, 27 June, barely eleven or twelve hours before the incident in which Marguerite Coste was poisoned. There had, however, been some preliminaries to the episode two days before, on the Thursday afternoon, when a man in a yellow and blue striped sailor suit approached an eighteen-year-old prostitute called Marianne Laverne. He told her how his master had come to town in order to enjoy himself with some girls, especially young girls. Then, on the next day, another young prostitute, twenty-year-old Marianette Laugier, was accosted in the street by the same manservant, who told her a similar story. On Saturday morning at eight o'clock, the girls, who each had rooms in a house on the rue d'Aubagne, were summoned by the man in the sailor suit to present themselves at what he described as a less conspicuous meeting place. This was the corner house where the rue d'Aubagne joined the rue des Capucins, and here, at ten o'clock, the girls duly found themselves waiting with two other prostitutes, twenty-year-old Rosette Coste and 23-year-old Mariette Borelly, in the latter's third-floor apartment.

In due course the manservant returned, escorting a man of aristocratic bearing who was dressed in a fine grey dress-coat lined with blue and who carried a sword and cane. The nobleman at once began to tease the girls, taking a handful of gold coins out of his pocket, announcing they were for them and that the girl who guessed how many he held in his hand would be his first partner. The youngest, Marianne Laverne, guessed correctly and so remained in the room with the nobleman and his valet while the rest of the girls were shooed out and the door locked.

There now began a laboured series of sexual antics as Marianne Laverne was made to lie face down on the bed next to the valet, while the nobleman used one hand to flog her, the other to 'excite his manservant'. Eventually the servant was dismissed from the room, at which point the nobleman produced a 'crystal snuff box encircled with gold' from a grey leather pouch. The box held tablets in the form of sweet aniseed balls, which he offered the girl, telling her to eat as many as she could since they would encourage her to grow 'windy'. She ate at least seven or eight, but declined when he asked her to eat more. Now he offered her a twenty-franc piece if she would allow his valet to 'take possession of her from behind', a suggestion which, she declared, she rejected completely.

By way of variation, the nobleman next took out a leather whip embellished with several large and small curved pins and ordered her to lash his buttocks. Marianne, however, could not bring herself to administer more than three half-hearted strokes with the 'cat-o'-nine-tails', and so the door was unlocked and a servant woman sent to purchase a heather broom. The young prostitute felt fewer qualms over striking him with this implement, and now managed to flog him as he cried out encouragement, calling for her to strike harder.

At this stage Marianne Laverne was beginning to feel faint and had grown aware of a distinct queasiness in her stomach. It was a relief when the nobleman chose to release her from the bedroom so that another girl might take her place. Mariette Borelly, the oldest prostitute, was next ushered in by the manservant and made to undress so that the orgy could be resumed. Again there were floggings administered and received, the nobleman carefully counting the strokes and using his knife to score up the totals on the mantelpiece. Again there was the manual stimulation of the manservant, and then an awkward moment of contrived abandon as the nobleman attempted to have sexual intercourse with the girl at the same time as he allowed himself to be sodomized by his valet.

In the bedroom the orgy thus pursued its repetitive progress, but in the kitchen Marianne Laverne was beginning to feel decidedly ill. She had pains in her abdomen and was trying to settle her disturbed stomach by drinking a basinful of water. When this brought no relief, she begged the servant woman to make her a cup of coffee.

Mariette Borelly had by this time served her turn, and then it was that of Rosette Coste, and finally that of Marianette Laugier. The last girl was not unnaturally already in a state of panic. At the sight of the whip, bloodstained by now, she made a bid to escape. The nobleman thereupon insisted that the first girl should also return to the bedroom, and both girls were offered sweets from the crystal snuff box. Marianette took some, but secretly dropped them on the floor; Marianne refused point blank to touch a single further one. Marianette, despite her efforts to escape, now found herself forced to watch as various indignities were forced upon Marianne, including additional experiments in what one modern author has termed 'Lego-sex'. At one point she was tied up and laid on her stomach on the bed with her dress tucked up behind while the nobleman, demanding to know whether 'the comforts had done anything for her', sniffed carefully at her buttocks.

Finally, the young prostitutes begged to be released, and, although the nobleman resorted to threats, the sequence of events seemed at last to have lost its impetus. The nobleman and his servant withdrew, leaving six francs each for the girls, and on the way out, after a whispered consultation, stopped to tip the servant woman who was regarding them with grave suspicion. In the bedroom, Marianette and Marianne both collapsed in tears, and within hours Marianne Laverne was rolling on her bed with abdominal cramps and vomiting blood followed by copious amounts of blackish material.

The *Lieutenant Général criminel* had no problems with discovering the identity of the nobleman. The servant woman, hovering in the kitchen, had recognized him. It had been the Marquis de Sade.

The identification was amply confirmed later, for the description of a nobleman in a grey dress-coat with a sword and gold-headed cane was to be instantly familiar to a series of witnesses. An actor-comedian, who had dined with the marquis on the Saturday evening immediately before the affair involving Marguerite Coste, stated that on that occasion the suspect had indeed been wearing marigold-coloured breeches. The nobleman's companion, the tall pock-marked man in a blue and yellow striped sailor suit, was likewise unhesitatingly identified as the Marquis de Sade's man-servant, Latour.

Chomel meanwhile sought out knife marks on the mantel-piece of the third-floor bedroom, and on the side of the chimney flue towards the window, a little to the right of the mirror, he found a series of numbers carved into the wall: 215, 179, 225, 240. The servant woman told him how, when the room was swept out, she had seen several small aniseed sweets entangled with the sweepings, but these were thrown out with the refuse. It was now four days since the incident, but Chomel still searched the room minutely. In a corner of the floor at the foot of the bed and at right angles to the wall he found a small square of folded paper which contained two small aniseed sweets.

Chomel now held enough evidence to suggest that at least two serious crimes had been committed. Under French law, sodomy was a criminal offence which might merit sentence of death for both the active and the passive partner, the savage statutory penalty being execution by burning at the stake. Rarely, if ever, was the extreme penalty carried through, but poisoning was also a capital offence, whether the victim died or recovered. The criminal act lay in administering the poison, and even if the victim managed to survive, this was not considered a defence in law. Poisoning was seen, in fact, as one of the most serious crimes, where a full severity of sentence might well be imposed. And it was on the suspected crime of poisoning that Chomel focused his attention.

Marguerite Coste's condition had been giving rise to considerable concern. Throughout Thursday, despite the soothing medicines and enemas, she continued to vomit, bringing up a thick yellowish bile. Although the abdominal pain seemed to be subsiding, she began to complain of discomfort in the region around her kidneys. The doctors from the Seneschal's Court were visiting her twice a day, but, afraid that their physical remedies were failing, she asked for a priest to be summoned. She made her confession on Thursday evening, though she was unable to take communion on account of the persistent vomiting. By Friday morning the doctors felt that her pulse was growing weaker. After midday, however, it became clear that the vomiting had subsided at last. She suffered a disturbed night, but on Saturday morning, although her tongue was still dry and her pulse feverish, the doctors felt sure she would recover.

The physicians prepared a full and careful account of her illness for the Seneschal's Court and were in no doubt that the disorder was caused by poisoning, declaring that her symptoms proceeded from a 'tearing and cauterization of the soft membrane of the stomach, this tearing and cauterization having been produced by some substance acrid and corrosive, probably in the tablets she had eaten'. They added that, although the patient's life was no longer in danger, she found herself in a most deplorable condition.

The life of the young prostitute, Marianne Laverne, had also been in peril, although it was only on Thursday that she was visited by the doctors. They found her lying in bed in her second-floor apartment in the rue d'Aubagne, still vomiting 'many substances black and bloody' and complaining of severe pain. Her pulse was agitated, her tongue moist and somewhat white. Beside her bed stood a large basin which contained much material, 'similar to swillings of flesh', with several streaks of fresh blood. On Friday she was feverish and still disturbed by vomiting and diarrhoea. When she drank, she experienced a burning sensation along the course of the throat and gullet, while there was a new pain in the region of her kidneys. By Saturday morning she was able to sleep a little while remaining feverish and troubled by discomfort and distention in her lower abdomen. She also experienced a 'burning heat from her urine'.

The doctors' report stated that Marianne Laverne was suffering 'from a slow excoriation of the passageways occasioned by the passage of some substance acrid and corrosive, whose action is also borne on the urinary passages', and that, while she was not quite out of danger, she was not yet beyond means of recovery. In the meantime, attempts were proceeding to identify the poison, which, it seemed certain, must have been concealed in the sweets. The first suspicion was that it was arsenic.

At ten o'clock in the morning of Thursday, 2 July, André Rimbaud and Jean-Baptiste Joseph Aubert, the official receivers of the community of apothecaries for the town of Marseille, had met the doctor and surgeon appointed to care for Marguerite Coste at Rimbaud's laboratory. Here they were to examine the sample of vomit which the *Lieutenant Général criminel* had recovered from Marguerite Coste's apartment.

Once the specimen was formally identified to the apothecary masters by Chomel himself, the official seal was broken and a dark-brown liquid emptied from the bottle. In the words of the original report, this was now 'guided and examined', the doctors quickly reaching the conclusion that the fatty, oily substances visible on the surface were the remains of medicines prescribed by the previous doctor and that the rest of the liquid consisted entirely of drinks and infusions taken by the patient.

Moving on to a more technical investigation, they began by heating it, but noted no visible change. The liquid was then distilled and produced an insipid water which smelt slightly putrid. The distillate, when added to spring water with a small quantity of copper solution, produced a mixture with a slight blue colour. When the mixture was allowed to stand overnight, no precipitation occurred and no deposit was formed.

The two small aniseed sweets discovered in Mariette Borelly's bedroom were found, under the microscope, to consist of grains of aniseed surrounded by artistically moulded coatings of sugar. A small particle of one of the sweets placed cautiously on the tongue produced no acrid sensation. When one of the sweets was burnt on the fire, no odour of arsenic could be observed. In a last attempt at analysis, the remaining fragment of sweet was dissolved in two drachms of hot water but failed to impart to it any colour whatsoever.

The apothecary masters, 'being unable to extend our experiments further because of the small quantities available', stated and reported that the 'liquid of the said bottle is not the substance which occasioned the vomiting of the patient and that the two comfits are not sufficient in quantity to subject them to experiments which would determine their nature and constitution'. Neither arsenic nor a corrosive sublimate nor, indeed, any other poisonous substance had been demonstrated. The apothecaries had been able to reach nothing except negative conclusions.

The failure to detect poison did not, however, deter the legal authorities. On Saturday, 4 July, as soon as he received medical reports declaring that both prostitutes were suffering from the effects of poison, Chomel presented his assembled evidence to the King's Procurator. A brisk dispatch at once ordered the arrest of both the Marquis de Sade and his manservant, Latour, while the fact that the last rites had been administered to Marguerite Coste caused the procurator some concern. Despite reassurances from the doctors, he was afraid that the original complainant and principal witness might die before the case could be brought to trial. He instructed that she was to be visited again and have her evidence taken in a signed deposition.

Inquiries showed that the nobleman and his valet had been staying at the Hôtel des Treize-Cantons, but that they had left Marseille early on Sunday morning, less than six hours after the visit to Marguerite Coste. By the time the hunt shifted forty-five miles to the north to the de Sade estate at La Coste, near Apt, and a mounted escort had been sent to arrest them, both the Marquis de Sade and Latour had fled to Savoy, which then came under the sovereignty of Sardinia.

Eight weeks later, on 3 September, despite the absence of both the marquis and his valet, the case was brought to trial. Marguerite Coste and Marianne Laverne, probably as a result of bribes, had retracted their statements, but even so the Marquis de Sade and Latour were found guilty of poisoning and sodomy. They were sentenced *in absentia*. Dressed in penitential shirts, with bare heads and feet, with ropes hung about their necks, with large yellow candles in their hands, they were to kneel before the door of the cathedral and make 'honourable amends' for their sins, asking pardon of God and the king. The Marquis de Sade was then to have his head struck off while Latour was to be hanged or strangled by the public executioner. Afterwards their bodies were to be burnt and the ashes scattered.

A scaffold was specially erected in the Place des Prêcheurs before the Church of Saint-Sauveur in Aix, and on 12 September 1772 the sentences were carried out. The authorities were obliged to substitute straw effigies, however, since the marquis and his manservant still contrived to avoid lending their presences.

Even before the trial began, rumours of the events at Marseille were spreading throughout the country. The name of the Marquis de Sade was already a byword for libertinage even in the profligate atmosphere of Louis XV's France. Reports of the scandals, debaucheries and perversions in which he had been involved had circulated widely and wildly, and accounts of the Marseille episode inevitably became luridly distorted. In one detail, however, they were remarkably uniform. They identified the poison concerned as having been Spanish fly, a 'love-drug' administered as an aphrodisiac. The *Mémoires secrets pour servir à l'histoire de la République des lettres en France* or the *Journal d'un observateur* (London, 1777) recorded the following version:

25th July 1772. This concerns Marseille where the Marquis de Sade . . . gave a ball to which he invited many people and in the dessert he had slipped chocolate drops so magnificent that many people ate them. There were plenty of them and hardly anybody abstained from them, but they had been mixed with Spanish flies. The virtue of this medicine is known. It was found that all those who had eaten it, burning with an immodest, passionate flame, were given over to all the excesses to which the most amorous passion carried them. The ball sank to the level of one of those licentious orgies renowned by the Romans: the most discreet ladies were not able to resist the passion which excited them . . . Many people have died of the excesses to which they were given in their dreadful lusts . . .

A different account was given in a pamphlet by J. A. Dulauré,

Collection de la liste des ci-devant Ducs, Marquis, Contes, Barons etc. (Paris, second year of liberty [1794]):

Together with his footman, he assembled some young courtesans at his house, made them take drinks, Spanish fly tablets and made them all excited and of an amorous disposition; he lit in their blood lecherous fires, to the extent that, devoured by an excessive sexual need, its satisfaction would become not only a need but an urgent remedy to an illness both real and dangerous. Instead of bringing the remedy the Marquis de Sade only presented it to enhance the desire; then he would gratify his filthy debauchery on his footman in the presence of the girls. These girls were dying . . .

The rumour of illicit poisoning by Spanish fly, with its fantasies of discreet women driven by irresistible passion into uterine frenzy, was one that refused to fade. In 1837, *La Revue de Paris* recounted the story as follows:

He returned to Marseille during the month of June, accompanied by a trusty servant whom he had prepared to be of use in his most criminal debauchery. He had provided for himself some chocolate drops in whose composition was included a strong dose of Spanish fly, that terrible and dangerous stimulant which produces such dreadful licentiousness in the nervous system. The two accomplices went together into a house of loose women where they supplied the wine, the drinks and the tablets which caused spasms: the effects of these tablets did not stop at laughter, lascivious dances and the distasteful symptoms of hysteria: one of these poor wretches that the stimulating drug had put into a similar state to that of the bacchantes of the olden days, threw herself through the window and fatally wounded herself, while others, semi-naked, indulged in more filthy prostitutions, in full view of the people who rushed in front of the house and who were shouting loudly and making distracted noises . . .

Spanish fly is one of the most ancient and least reputable drugs known to man. It has been in use for at least two thousand years since Hippocrates described its application in treating dropsy. By the end of the seventeenth century, Groeneveldt, in *De tuto cantharidum in medicina usu internol* (London, 1698), was referring to it as indispensable in the treatment of bladder and kidney infections, stone, strangury, dropsy and certain venereal diseases. When applied to the skin it caused pain and blistering, and a use was found for it as a counter-irritant for such painful conditions as sciatica and pleurisy.

Yet it is for its reputation as an aphrodisiac that Spanish fly has continued to fascinate the popular mind. Administered orally in minute quantities, the drug causes an irritation of the kidneys and bladder, an aching in the pelvis and the frequent and uncomfortable voiding of small amounts of urine, passed with a sensation of scalding or burning. These pelvic discomforts were thought to enhance a woman's awareness of her genitalia and, by proximity, to arouse and inflame a desire, even an urgent need, for sexual intercourse. In the male, the same irritation of the urinary tract was expected to stimulate a similar urgency of desire, while prolonged and powerful erections were credited to the drug's influence. Its hazards for either sex, however, included the fact that it can lead to haemorrhages in the kidneys and bladder, and even the suppression of urine, while in the male priapism occurs only with toxic and maybe fatal doses.

The name of the drug came from the insect which supplied it. The Spanish fly, *Cantharis vesicatoria*, is a handsome green beetle which produces blisters on the skin if handled. It is found in southern France and Spain, clustered on privet or such trees as the ash and elder. By tradition, the beetles were gathered before sunrise while still torpid and unable to fly, the collectors veiling their faces and hands before shaking them down on to cloths laid on the ground. The drug was then prepared as a powder made by pounding the dried corpses of the insects, or sometimes as a tincture produced by dissolving this powder in alcohol, or else as a vinegar by percolation with acetic acid and water.

Aphrodisiac sweets were made by impregnating sugared sweets, and as such were widely used under the name *pilles galantes*. They were also sometimes called *pastilles de Richelieu*, so well known was it that the Duc de Richelieu administered them to his mistresses, and it was said that Madame du Barry referred to them as *pastilles de sérail* (pastilles of the seraglio), using them on herself, or at least administering them to young women to prepare them for their sexual duties with the ageing Louis XV.

It was in 1810 that a French chemist, Roviquet, succeeded in isolating the active principle of the drug, a chemical present in the ovaries, soft tissues and blood of the beetle, which was subsequently called cantharidin. The various documents in the case make it clear that senior officials in Marseille and Provence suspected Spanish fly had been used in the Marquis de Sade's *cause célèbre*, but the apothecary masters could hardly have been expected to identify a chemical not yet discovered.

The sweets offered to the prostitutes of Marseille seem, in fact, to have been an enterprising attempt at polypharmacy. The core of each one consisted of a grain of aniseed, and aniseed enjoyed a wide reputation as a carminative: that is to say, it was a drug which led to the production and expulsion of excessive flatus from the bowel. One of Chomel's witnesses, another prostitute familiar with the unusual tastes of the marquis, explained that he administered aniseed to produce windiness in his partner, so that she might 'explode in his mouth', *péter en gueule* being a specialized perversion in which the mouth is used to catch a fart. Hence, by surrounding the aniseed in a coating of sugar impregnated with Spanish fly, de Sade clearly aimed at obtaining a double effect.

The house-physician at St James's Hospital, Balham, was summoned from bed by an emergency call from the medical ward at six o'clock on the morning of Tuesday, 27 April 1954. The 27-year-old typist, admitted to hospital the night before, had suddenly collapsed. According to the night staff, she became stiff before relaxing and finally lapsing into unconsciousness. When the house-physician arrived she was deeply comatose with a weak flickering pulse and a blood pressure so low it could not be measured. An hour afterwards she was dead.

Five hours later a post-mortem examination showed she had beyond doubt died from a corrosive poison. The naked-eye findings were consistent with the changes which Professor Rimmington had thought would occur if his suspicions were correct: they were those to be expected in cantharidin poisoning.

At University College Hospital, the condition of the younger typist was also desperate. At nine that morning, after having passed no urine for sixteen hours, she was catheterized and passed a few ounces of heavily bloodstained urine. She was sliding into a state of intense circulatory shock, and despite determined efforts at resuscitation her condition continued rapidly downhill. She died at 4.40 in the afternoon, barely twenty-four hours after admission. A post-mortem showed findings similar to those in the older girl.

The police now knew what they were looking for, and back at the premises of the chemical wholesaler's in Euston Road, a direct question brought a direct answer. Yes, one of the pharmacists confirmed, the company did retain a small stock of cantharidin, the total amount being kept in a small bottle in a glass cupboard in his own office. A quick check suggested that a small amount had gone missing, later measurement showing that 40 grains (2·5 grams) of powder had been removed.

Even more interestingly, the pharmacist remarked on how the police were not the first people in the week to ask about the chemical. There had been an inquiry within the firm on the morning of that fatal Monday, when he was somewhat surprised to have the office manager come into his room and ask whether they stocked cantharidin. The pharmacist took the bottle from the cupboard to show it to him and asked why he needed it. A neighbour, the manager explained, was hoping to get hold of some since he kept rabbits and was having trouble getting them to breed. The pharmacist stated that he certainly could not part with any of the crystals, pointing out that it was a dangerous drug. It apparently came as a surprise to the office manager to know that cantharidin was a schedule one poison, but he accepted the refusal philosophically, saying: 'Oh well, if that is the case, I don't want it!' But then a woman clerk had remembered how she thought it odd, when she went into the pharmacist's room later on, just before lunch, to find the office manager in there by himself.

The future of the investigation now lay with the Metropolitan Police Laboratory at New Scotland Yard and its highly skilled and eminent director, Dr L. C. Nickolls. Lewis Nickolls was the analytical chemist who helped to start Britain's first forensic laboratory at Hendon in 1935. He moved from there to become founding director of the North-Eastern Forensic Laboratory in Wakefield, and eventually, in 1951, took over the direction of the laboratory at New Scotland Yard. His experience of scientific criminal investigation encompassed the unravelling of over a thousand murders, including those committed by John Reginald Christie at 10 Rillington Place. But Dr Nickolls now found himself confronting precisely the problem which had defeated the apothecary masters of Marseille. The advances in knowledge and technique brought by an interval of a century and three quarters still seemed scarcely sufficient for the task of solving it.

Cantharidin is a comparatively simple organic compound which occurs as colourless, odourless crystals. These glisten in light yet give no colour reactions and cannot be detected by any simple chemical test. The old powdered preparations of Spanish fly could be identified by using a microscope to show the characteristic fragments of insect in the powder. Identifying pure cantharidin was still a much more difficult task, and after a series of preliminary experiments Lewis Nickolls concluded that there were only three ways in which he could arrive at a positive identification for cantharidin: by its melting point; by the X-ray diffraction pattern obtained from its crystals; and by the standard observation that, when cantharidin is applied to human skin, pain and blistering are produced.

Dr Nickolls first carefully inspected the debris collected from the desk surfaces in the main office. The dust from the office manager's desk, he found, contained minute, colourless crystals, while the X-ray diffraction pattern obtained from them matched exactly that given by cantharidin crystals from the small stock bottle in the pharmacist's cupboard. Thus there was no doubt that, at some point, a minute quantity of cantharidin had, indeed, been spilt on the manager's desk.

Now he turned his attention to the scissors found in the manager's desk drawer. The smears on the scissor blades in fact produced a confused and complicated X-ray diffraction pattern, but careful comparisons showed this simply to consist of two superimposed patterns: that given by coconut-icing and that obtained from cantharidin. The material clinging to the blades of the scissors consisted of a mixture of coconut-icing and cantharidin crystals.

The most difficult part of Dr Nickolls's investigations was, however, yet to come: the examination of two groups of biological specimens. The first group consisted of samples of vomit from each girl, the second of organs and material removed *post mortem*. He could not even attempt to identify cantharidin before each specimen had been subjected to a long and complex process to separate out every trace of the drug from the biological mixture in which it was suspended. A prolonged sequence of filtrations, extractions and precipitations eventually produced an oily residue from the samples of vomit. Ultimately, from this residue, by a process known as micro-sublimation, he produced the characteristic rectangular plates of pure cantharidin crystals.

Yet while he could now show that both typists had swallowed cantharidin, the organs and tissues themselves defeated any precise analysis. Try as he might, he could obtain no crystalline residue free from the all-pervading fatty acids. Only the simple biological test of applying an extract of specimen material to the human skin was going to provide the final proof, and once again he needed to work his way through a series of preliminary experiments, using pure cantharidin to establish the appearance and extent of blistering which a standard amount of the drug might be expected to produce. Extracts of vomit cautiously applied to the skin now produced typical blisters, and by measuring and comparing these against those produced in his control experiment he found that he could estimate the concentration of cantharidin in the vomit. Using the same technique, he was also able to prove that cantharidin was present in the body tissues.

At last Dr Nickolls felt able to make a confident and precise statement: each girl had been poisoned by cantharidin, each receiving a dose of between one and two grains (65–130 milligrams), though the 27-year-old had taken the slightly larger dose of the two. The procedures used had been tested by adding measured amounts of pure cantharidin to post-mortem specimens and tissues, the completeness and accuracy of the extractions and estimations being checked at every step. The Metropolitan Police Laboratory had managed to isolate, identify and measure a drug present in tissues as a concentration of approximately 0·00015 per cent.

A point which escaped almost all the press and legal commentators at the time, but which would have been perfectly well known to Dr Nickolls, was that applying cantharidin to human skin is at best a hazardous procedure. The drug can penetrate unbroken skin, with toxic, if not fatal, results. Only a year before, in 1953, a keen 43-year-old fisherman had managed to obtain some cantharidin, believing it would attract fish. After shaking up the powder with water, he stopped the mouth of the bottle with his thumb, and then, within minutes, unfortunately pricked his thumb with one of his fish-hooks. Within half an hour the fisherman was ill, within three days dead. To quote the dry comment of the *British Medical Journal*, any 'subject who submitted himself to the blister test in the interests of justice displayed admirable courage'.

The office manager had been in University College Hospital for almost three days when, early on Thursday morning, 29 April, Detective Superintendent John Jamieson approached him in the ward. The police had insisted that he should not be told of the typists' deaths, and, when Superintendent Jamieson informed him that they were dead and that it was believed they had died from cantharidin poisoning, he broke down, crying out: 'Oh my God! Why didn't somebody tell me!' Invited to go to Albany Street Police Station, he replied: 'I will do anything.'

In the car he appeared to be in a state of shock, saying over and over: 'I am to blame! I don't know what made me do it.' At the police station he needed to be supported as he walked from the car, and almost half-carried up the stairs to the interview room. Here he turned to his interviewers and said: 'I have been a fool! Let me tell you the story.'

By 9.30 that morning the manager was embarked on his second statement in the affair. He confessed that the tales he told the pharmacist about his neighbour and the rabbits had been untrue. It all went back to when he left Singapore in 1946, having served there in the Royal Army Service Corps. When the troopship home called at Aden, he listened as other soldiers discussed Spanish fly and the way it stimulated sexual feelings. He had given this no further thought until about three weeks ago when Spanish fly was mentioned in the office and he learnt for the first time that the medical name for the drug was cantharidin. He then, during stock-taking, noticed cantharidin on the inventories and decided to try to obtain some.

After the chemist inadvertently showed him where the drug was stored, he found the chance to be alone in the chemist's office and poured some cantharidin crystals into an empty wages packet. Acting out of curiosity, he had tipped a small quantity of crystals on to his desk top to inspect them. He had no idea what happened to those scattered crystals, but at lunch time he bought some coconut-icing from the sweet shop and came back to the office. He emptied the coconut-icing from its bag on to his desk, dividing it up, giving some pieces to the girls and eating some himself. He could only think that it was in this way that the coconut-icing became contaminated. He had not thought to look for the crystals scattered on the desk and he had not deliberately given the crystals to the girls in any form.

As soon as the statement was laboriously written out in long-hand and duly signed, he was shown the scissors from his desk drawer. All at once he announced: 'I have been thinking a lot about this. My mother always told me to tell the truth.' As he made his third and final statement, he began: 'I now wish to say that I took a little cantharidin from the wages envelope and put it into the coconut-icing with the scissors you have shown me . . .'

The manager had deliberately prepared a piece of coconut-icing for the older girl, 'so that she would want intercourse with me'. 'We were very fond of each other,' he said, 'but she was always putting me off.' He persistently denied knowing how the younger typist, the beauty queen, could have come to take any of the adulterated coconut-icing.

In speaking of the older typist, he described her as a very gentle person, an intelligent but solitary girl who made few friends and had very few boyfriends. She had worked in his office for several years, proving herself to be a quiet, quick, yet thorough assistant who could be relied upon when things were rushed. At first, so she told him later, she had felt an intense dislike for him, but, after a quarrel which culminated with him telling her off, a discreet friendship had sprung up between them.

They sat, during the working day, almost facing one another across the long office desk, but, when they began to meet over coffee, would leave and return to the office separately. He found her a sympathetic listener who seemed to demand nothing but friendship. On birthdays or such special occasions as Christmas Eve, they would buy each other small gifts and he would take her to a Lyons corner house. Once he bought her a brooch set with a large circular blue stone. They would meet each morning for a cup of coffee on the way to work, exchanging a good-morning kiss before parting so as to arrive separately at the office door.

In due course, in what was probably an instinctive attempt to readjust the nature of the relationship, he invited his friend home for tea to meet his wife and family. The wife saw in her no great beauty, but a quiet girl who dressed simply yet smartly in blacks and greens and said how much she enjoyed being in what she called a really happy home. She was invited to return and brought presents for the children. She offered to sit with the children so that the manager and his wife could get out together at weekends. Before long she was a regular visitor, spending almost every weekend at their home, arriving on Friday evening and leaving for work on Monday morning.

She was not, the wife felt, the sort of girl a wife would need to get jealous over. She knew she was always confiding her troubles to her husband, and that the two often had lunch together, but that was simply business. While the girl seemed fonder of him than was perhaps wise, her husband could be trusted to handle matters with tact and discretion.

Yet, for the manager himself, the situation grew hopelessly involved, the emotional pressures intense. Four years earlier he had given the girl a rose that his wife had placed in his buttonhole. Now she produced it, carefully pressed, dried and preserved between the pages of a book. He found that she excited him and that he wanted her. Once, he claimed, he persuaded her to make love furtively in the office but she had not enjoyed it. Her closeness and gentle affection were both tantalizing and evasive. 'She kept saying she would let me do it next time,' he told the police. 'When the next time came I made up my mind to give her cantharidin to stimulate her desire for me.'

When Superintendent Jamieson told him he would be charged with causing the typist's death, the manager exclaimed: 'Oh dear God! What an awful thing I have done! What about the other girl?' As he was escorted back to the detention room, he became agitated and distressed, calling out the older girl's name and crying over and over: 'Oh, I did not kill you!'

The following day, dressed in a brown suit and a black tie, the manager appeared in the dock at Clerkenwell Magistrates Court. He was allowed to sit during the proceedings and stared straight ahead as he was remanded in custody on a charge of manslaughter.

On 18 June he was brought to trial before the Lord Chief Justice, Lord Goddard, at the Central Criminal Courts, where he pleaded guilty to the manslaughter of both typists. It was accepted that he had meant to administer the drug only to the older girl and that the poisoning of the younger typist was caused by 'an incredible piece of carelessness'. His own illness was put down to a tiny amount of cantharidin being accidentally brushed on to his lips and cheek by his contaminated fingers after he prepared the coconut-icing. His defence counsel admitted he had not been able to obtain any coherent instructions from his client, describing the manager as 'physically and mentally something like a wreck'. In his brief address, counsel was able to tell the court that the manager's wife had forgiven her husband and intended to stand by him. He rounded off his remarks by trying to suggest, as a mitigating factor, that to some degree it was the manager's ignorance of the 'ways of wickedness' which had launched the tragedy.

The Lord Chief Justice, however, described it as the most distressing case of manslaughter in all his experience and sentenced the office manager to five years' imprisonment.

*

The Marquis de Sade never had any intention of avoiding the 'ways of wickedness' during the course of his life. As an atheist, he denied the authority of God and man in all its forms, and partly as a result of this standpoint found himself spending most of his last thirty-six years either in prison or in a lunatic asylum. He wrote copiously and indiscriminately, producing plays and political pamphlets as well as such classic erotic novels as *Justine* and *The Hundred and Twenty Days at Sodom*, the latter cataloguing man's sexual perversions to a total of six hundred. He foretold the coming of the French Revolution, welcomed it when it broke and at one point only narrowly escaped the guillotine. He acknowledged that women's rights to sexual pleasure were equal to men's when he wrote: 'If we admit . . . that all women should submit to our desires, surely we ought also to allow them to fully satisfy their own.'

He gave his name to the term 'sadism' in modern psychology and has his place in European intellectual history. He wilfully opened doors on to the dark corners of the human mind where love, desire and cruelty often overlap. Yet in his urge to live through extremes of experience in life as well as in his imagination he was driven by a demon in his loins that would not let him rest and which provoked such incidents as that with the prostitutes in Marseille. He ended his days, not as the Byronic monster of his myth, but as an obese little white-haired old gentleman, much tormented by gout, rheumatism and eye trouble, though at least allowed by the enlightened director of the Charenton asylum, where he was confined, to write and produce plays in which he cast his fellow-inmates.

The marquis died at seventy-four in 1814, having left in his will instructions for the disposal of his body that have a certain stoical dignity. He asked that it be taken by cart to the family estate at La Coste and there buried without ceremony in a small wood close to the *château*. Acorns were to be strewn in the freshly turned soil so that, as the coppice thickened, all traces of his grave and of his memory would disappear from the face of the earth and the minds of men. In the event the wishes of the arch-atheist were denied and he was interred with Christian rites in the asylum cemetery.

Some years after his death, his son, discovering that a universal biography was nearing the letter S, wrote to the biographer begging him not to include his father's name.

The office manager and his wife sold their respective stories to the Sunday newspapers.

Chapter 10

The Contagion and the Rose

The Lying-In Division of the Boston Hospital for Women, associated as it is with Harvard Medical School, is one of the world's most advanced institutions in the care of expectant, puerperal and post-natal mothers. In terms of technological standing, it can fairly be said to be second to none. Yet a microbe of the wrong sort may, from time to time, breach the defences of even the best-run medical institution. Any sign of illness in a mother fresh from the delivery room is likely to attract close attention, especially if she runs a fever, since a high temperature is not a general or natural feature of giving birth. It is usually a sign that something has gone amiss with protecting a woman at the point in her life where she is particularly vulnerable to infection. This may not have been understood a century ago, when the malady known variously as 'lying-in fever', 'childbed fever' or 'puerperal fever' was thought of as a commonplace if haphazardly occurring corollary to the whole business of becoming a mother. In those days, many physicians were resigned to losing a proportion of mothers in their care to a contagion which seemed to strike out of the very air. That particular angel of death has, during the present century, come to be regarded as largely banished from hospital wards and the broad experience of doctors and midwives, though this is not to say it is no longer capable of causing alarm with a distant flap of its wings.

When, fourteen hours after the delivery of her child, a mother in the Boston Lying-In Division was found to have a temperature of just over 101°F, her doctor took an alert interest. It was three o'clock in the afternoon of 24 April 1965, and there was no need for immediate concern, though the situation was one which should be watched while routine tests were put in motion. By the evening of the following day her temperature had risen to 103°F, and apart from the fever, a general sense of being unwell and a loss of appetite, she felt chilled and had a vague discomfort in her pelvic region. Results of the tests were awaited but were not yet available.

On the 26th, two more mothers developed temperatures, as did three on the next day and one more on the day after that. Up to this point, each mother was being treated as an individual case problem by her own doctor, but now a fresh dimension was introduced as matters moved towards a climax. No less than seven mothers, all delivered of their children on the 29th, duly showed similar symptoms.

The Boston Lying-In Division needed to face the implication that it was having to deal with an epidemic of what was formerly a woman's most ruthless post-natal enemy: puerperal sepsis. The irony was that the hospital was known world-wide for its pioneering work in obstetric safety standards. Its research programmes had produced dramatic advances in knowledge of the development of the human embryo and the function of the placenta. Within its walls, the exchange transfusion had been perfected for saving the lives of babies affected at birth by an incompatibility between their parents' blood groups (the so-called rhesus incompatibility). The institution braced itself as the patients became, for the most part, extremely ill, several showing a full set of the classic symptoms of puerperal fever, including chills with fever, flushed cheeks, glazed eyes, exaggerated elation of mood, distended abdomens and acute tenderness in the ovaries and Fallopian tubes. It was already the worst recorded outbreak in any American hospital since 1927, when twenty-four patients at the Sloan Hospital in New York developed infections, nine mothers and two infants dying as a consequence.

Hippocrates, 'the father of medicine', noted down several case histories of women who met distressing deaths from puerperal pestilence in the fifth century BC. Among these in *Epidemics*, Book I, xii, is described a seventeen-year-old who developed a fever shortly after bearing a son.

To start with she suffered from thirst, nausea and a slight ache in the heart; her tongue was parched and the bowels were disordered . . . She did not sleep.

Second day: slight rigors, a high fever, a small amount of cold sweating about the head . . .

Fourth day: all symptoms more pronounced . . .

Seventh day: rigors, high fever, thirst, much tossing about. Towards evening, cold sweating all over and became chilled; the extremities were cold and did not get warm again. Further rigors during the night; extremities still would not get warm; no sleep and some delirium . . . [*Hippocratic Writings*, edited by G. E. R. Lloyd, translated by J. Chadwick and W. N. Mann, Pelican Classics, 1978]

On the ninth day, her symptoms abated, but on the day following, her 'fever increased in a paroxysm' and thereafter her condition rapidly deteriorated until she met her end on the fourteenth day of her illness.

Over the centuries after Hippocrates, other doctors left accounts of cases of 'childbed fever', but, while the condition was known and rightly feared, it did not have too common an incidence. There were no clues to its cause, no known satisfactory treatment. Some mothers who became infected died, while others happily recovered.

In the course of time, and during the eighteenth century in particular, the lying-in hospitals became established features of the cities of Europe. These institutions were, like the Westminster Lying-In Hospital opened in April 1767, designed for the wives of the poor and needy, though the Westminster wards also admitted single women 'such as are deserted, and in deep distress, to save them from Despair, and the lamentable Crimes of Suicide and Child Murder'. Formed for the best and most benevolent of reasons, the lying-in hospitals nevertheless introduced a new chapter in the history of this septic fever which at times killed as many as 20 per cent of the women they had been set up to rescue from suffering. The fever in fact became the major cause of death in newly delivered mothers.

As women naturally began to fear their confinements in the lying-in institutions, the illness continued to preserve the secret of its mode of attack. Although it did seem at times to be carried by the air, it was also noticed how it could apparently attach itself to certain doctors or midwives, who sometimes lost custom as their reputations grew for burying the mothers in their care. No one knew what it was or where it came from, though some thoughtful members of the medical profession, such as Charles White, a notable man-midwife and surgeon of Manchester in the later eighteenth century, did meet with success in preventing and treating the disease. White was in advance of his contemporaries in seeing it as possibly a contagion of some kind, and far in advance of them in advocating basic hygiene, clean bed-linen and fresh air at a time when none of these fancy notions was established in medical practice.

Certain individual spirits were less inclined than others to accept the heavily prevailing view that there was nothing to be done, but the prevailing view held its ground for the best part of a further century. In the words of an eminent American obstetrician, Professor Meigs of Philadelphia, expressed in 1842, puerperal fever was no more than 'a group of diverse inflammations within the belly'. The person who first made it his business to marshal the known facts was a doctor from Boston who became professor of physiology and anatomy, as well as dean of the medical faculty, at Harvard University. His name was Oliver Wendell Holmes and he was better known to the public as a literary figure, the poet and essayist who was author of *The Autocrat of the Breakfast Table*.

His essay 'The Contagiousness of Puerperal Fever' was originally published in the *New England Quarterly Journal of Medicine and Surgery* in April 1843. It was a medical pronouncement of the first importance, his intention having been, he wrote later, 'to show that women had often died in childbed, poisoned by their medical attendants'. Here was the crux of the matter, for it involved a controversial thesis which the bulk of established medical opinion found untenable and impertinent. The author himself came under instant counter-attack, such authorities as Professor Meigs pouring a mocking scorn on the ideas he set out to promote. Meigs took the view that doctors were gentlemen and that 'a gentleman's hands are clean'.

Yet Holmes had argued his case with a combination of passionate concern and literary eloquence. The evidence he assembled from both medical literature and personal testimony was formidable and utterly clear-sighted. In example after example he described how the infection had sprung up in the footsteps of one physician, nurse or midwife or another as they passed between existing cases or from autopsy room to lying-in chamber. It seemed incredible, he wrote, 'that any should be found too prejudiced or ignorant to accept the solemn truth knelled into their ears by the funeral bells from both sides of the ocean – the plain conclusion that the physician and the disease entered, hand in hand, into the chamber of the unsuspecting patient'. He was contributing no original research, and did not claim to know or say of what the 'contagion' consisted. The lives of patients were, to him, more important than professional reputations, and he wished only to express the facts staring them in the face. He ended by defining puerperal fever as a *'private pestilence* in the sphere of a single physician' which should be looked on 'not as a misfortune but a crime; and in the knowledge of such occurrences, the duties of the practitioner to his profession, should give way to his paramount obligations to society'.

Some among Holmes's contemporaries, in Britain as well as the United States, were willing to take note, but overall it was his opponents who held sway. The journal in which his paper appeared only survived a few issues and, though the ripples of its influence continued to spread, Holmes was naturally aware that it was the Meigses of this world who all too often held the ears of medical students just at the stage where young men's attitudes were most open and formative. When, in 1855, he reissued his essay, retitling it 'Puerperal Fever as a Private Pestilence', he included a special appeal to student minds in the commentary which he added. Nothing in the intervening twelve years had lessened his conviction; quite the reverse. There was, by now, a tone of indignation, even of desperation, in his response to the bitter attacks he had suffered.

No man [he wrote] makes a quarrel with me over the counterpane that covers a mother, with her new-born infant at her breast! There is no epithet in the vocabulary of slight and sarcasm that can reach my personal sensibilities in such a controversy.

Towards the close he commented:

I am too much in earnest for either humility or vanity, but I do entreat those who hold the keys of life and death, to listen to me also for this once. I ask no personal favour; but I beg to be heard, in behalf of the women whose lives are at stake, until some stronger voice shall plead for them.

. . . Let the men who mould opinions look to it; if there is any voluntary blindness, any interested oversight, any culpable negligence, even, in such a matter, and the facts shall reach the public ear; the pestilence-carrier of the lying-in-chamber must look to God for pardon, for man will never forgive him.

In his list of additional references, Holmes included one from the Continent concerning a method of disinfection proposed by a M. 'Semmeliveis', alleged to have achieved a sudden and great decrease of mortality in lying-in wards. This was an obvious misspelling for the name of a young Hungarian doctor, Ignaz Philipp Semmelweis, who originally took up an appointment at the Vienna Lying-In Hospital in 1844. Circumstances had left Semmelweis, during his first couple of years at the hospital, with time to pursue his own line of research into the pathological causes for the deaths of women during or following childbirth. One observation in particular struck him forcibly. A high mortality rate in a lying-in hospital was accepted as normal, so how did it come about that, in the Vienna hospital, where the wards were split into two divisions, the divisions showed a marked relative discrepancy in fatalities?

An earlier director to the Lying-In Hospital, Professor Boer, had introduced Charles White's methods into his regime, against opposition but with markedly good results. His successor, Professor Klein, lost no time in putting the clock back when he took office in 1822. Under Klein, the fluctuating death-rate rose sharply from an annual average of 1·3 per cent, and continued to fluctuate, reaching, in bad months, figures as high as 29·3 per cent. In 1840, however, the administration of obstetric work was split into two divisions, the first being exclusively for the teaching of medical students and the second being for the training of midwives. It was between these divisions that the discrepancy occurred, and Semmelweis plotted out the relative death-rates over a five-year period. In the first division, mortality ran at 9·9 per cent, whereas in the second it did not reach above 3·9 per cent. The mothers themselves were well aware of the odds against them should they be so unfortunate as to come under the care of the doctors and their students in division one and often begged and wept not to be admitted.

So far as theories on the origins of puerperal fever went, the opinions of the 'contagionists', backed in America by Oliver Wendell Holmes, had not on the Continent gained the measure of practical ground which they held in both Britain and the United States. European obstetricians were unshakeably convinced that the disease resulted from an atmospheric influence or miasma tantamount to an act of God. Semmelweis's figures forced a search for other theses, since there seemed to be no reason why an incipient miasma should not affect one set of Viennese wards as much as the other.

Differences in diet, in ventilation, in treatment, even in the weather were all advanced as likely causes. More remote than these was the idea that it had something to do with certain 'metamorphoses' produced by the original conceiving sperm. 'Wounded modesty' was also seen as a possible explanation: a response to being examined by male students as opposed to midwives. An official inquiry, set up by Professor Klein, became quite convinced that the cause must be 'injuries to the genital organs', students being rougher than midwives in their approach. Semmelweis remained highly sceptical of all such provisional 'solutions'. In any case, reducing the numbers of students as well as of examinations produced no change whatsoever in mortality rates where the supposed ham-fistedness of students was concerned.

It was at this point that fate intervened with an object lesson when a professor of medical jurisprudence, who also happened to be a close friend of Semmelweis, suffered a slight injury as a surgical knife being used in a post-mortem examination accidentally pricked his finger. This minor wound swiftly developed into an acute and fatal case of blood-poisoning, and Semmelweis was instantly struck by the set of parallels between his friend's illness and a case of puerperal fever. The line of reasoning for which he had been searching stood all at once illuminated in a beam of clear light. The dead professor had, through a small wound, been infected by contaminated matter from a dissected corpse. A woman who gives birth temporarily carries inside her the equivalent of an extensive wound where the placenta has separated from the womb. The students came, as often as not, direct from the autopsy room to examine the mothers, and hence carried the spores of death in the form of infectious cadaveric particles.

The next development was that Semmelweis startled and outraged his students by imposing an inflexible rule that they scrub their hands in a solution of lime chloride before even so much as touching their patients. The results were dramatic. Over two years the death-rates on the students' wards were reduced from about one in six to one in a hundred. The pity of it was that Professor Klein, enthusiast for medical infallibility, still held the reins of power in Vienna and had suffered no mortal wound in the autopsy room. He made it his business to ensure that Semmelweis's contract was not extended after 1849.

Wherever he worked thereafter, however, Semmelweis applied his doctrine. It was unfortunate that he lacked the gift of clarity with words that Holmes possessed, and positively hated writing. He therefore relied on others to spread the news of his methods, and when in 1861 he at last produced his life-work, *The Etiology, Concept and Prophylaxis of Childbed Fever*, it turned out to be an impossibly long, densely and confusingly argued book, quarrelsome and difficult in tone. He had seen the truth so clearly, yet the disagreements continued to rage between those who supported and those who rejected his views. The opposition, firm in its standpoint of medical orthodoxy and reinforced by a strong emotional reluctance to accept that it could be doctors who carried the disease to patients, remained powerful and dominant. As the controversy pursued its course, Semmelweis himself began to suffer from periods of mental instability. He was admitted to a lunatic asylum on 1 August 1865, and died there twelve days later. It was noticed he had cut his hand, probably during one of the last gynaecological operations he performed, and the cut was infected. His leading contribution to medical science had been to recognize puerperal fever as a form of septicaemia or blood-poisoning, and this was the very infection which killed him.

The obituary notices of Austria and Germany were scant and dismissive of the 'Hungarian crank', and it was only during the years following his death that his vision came to be vindicated as advances began to be made in microbiology and the recognition of the part which germs played in infection. Eventually the great French chemist Louis Pasteur demonstrated in 1879 that the bacteria which he found in

post-natal discharges were also responsible for causing puerperal fever. The story was told of how, during an academic
discussion, a speaker expounding on what were traditionally
regarded as the causes of childbed fever was interrupted by
Pasteur with the words: 'None of these things causes an
epidemic. It is nursing and medical staff who carry the
microbe from an infected woman to a healthy one.' The
original speaker ventured to suggest that such an organism
would never be found. Pasteur replied by going to the
blackboard and drawing a set of small circles in a characteristic
chain-link formation. 'There you are!' he said. 'That's what
it's like!' The opposition was finally quelled.

In 1965, the micro-organism responsible for the outbreak
at the Boston Lying-In Division was promptly identified. It
was a germ that science classified and labelled as *beta*-
hemolytic streptococcus group A (T type 28), a species
thought to have played a major role in the childbed fever
epidemics of the past. Now, however, it was attempting to do
its worst in an establishment famous for its obstetric care,
which had, moreover, been, in 1847, the first maternity unit
in the United States to offer anaesthesia to help women in
labour. The counter-attack launched against the intruding
microbe was formidable in terms of both tactics and armoury.
The hospital authorities faced two imperative tasks: to stop
it in its tracks and to establish its source and ensure its
elimination.

All non-urgent operations and inductions of labour were
cancelled. Apart from quarantining and treating the sick
mothers, every new patient was placed on a carefully planned
regime of antibiotics. The medical staff underwent a similar
preventive routine, and the entire hospital personnel, to a
total of 800, was comprehensively screened. Throat swabs
were taken and checked and no skin breaks, however minute,

were neglected. A panel of leading experts was called into consultation.

Quarantining had been put into force on 29 April. Despite this and the massive, strenuous campaign of prevention and investigation, to the dismay of the authorities six further cases occurred during the week which followed. These were, however, the last, and the tension began to relax. In all, twenty mothers and one infant had been infected, but none of them was lost and all began to make a recovery, aided by the most recent advances in antibiotic therapy. Science had won the day, but the question remained of how the potentially lethal infection made its entrance in the first place.

There was a mass of data on patients and medical staff to be sifted, but two facts emerged. First, each of the women affected had been in the recovery room – but then most newly delivered mothers passed a spell in the recovery room. Second, over half the infected mothers had been attended during labour by the same anaesthetist. The anaesthetist had, by coincidence, gone off duty for a few days after the epidemic started, but as soon as he took his place in the screening process it was found that he bore two tiny scratches, one on his hand and one on his chin. These arose from his having recently pruned his roses, but were so insignificant he had paid them no attention; yet when a culture was made from material taken from under the scabs, it was found to carry streptococci of a type matching the infections present in a majority of the mothers. It was not even that he had played any active obstetric role during the processes of delivery, though he had in the natural course of events held each mother's hand to give comfort and reassurance while anaesthetic was administered.

The episode provided a salutary reminder, not only of what could lie in wait for mothers should vigilance ever be relaxed in their delivery rooms and wards, but also of the battles which had needed to be fought and won to make childbirth as safe a process today as it has ever been in human history. Only a hundred years before, obstetric science was still by and large in its dark ages, though the forces of light and reason had found their heroes: the sharp-penned champion of the cause, Oliver Wendell Holmes, and the awkward martyr-saint, Ignaz Philipp Semmelweis, posthumously hailed as 'the saviour of mothers'.

'Others had cried out with all their might against the terrible evil before I did,' wrote Holmes in 1893, the year before his death. '. . . But I think I shrieked my warning louder and longer than any of them . . . before the little army of microbes had moved up to support my position.' Semmelweis had remarked more sadly that, if it was not to be vouchsafed to him to see with his own eyes that happy time when the truth concerning the causes of puerperal fever was acknowledged and acted upon, then 'the conviction that such a time must inevitably sooner or later arrive will cheer my dying hour'. For the profession, the lesson never to be ignored was that the happy time came round despite, not because of, a consensus of eminent opinion.

Chapter 11

The Head that Wore a Crown

In 1968 in the anatomical museum of the University of Edinburgh, a Danish doctor who was a leading authority on skeletal archaeology stood confronting the plaster cast of the skull of a medieval monarch. The doctor's name was Vilhelm Møller-Christensen, and his part in the story began in the 1930s when, as a general practitioner in the town of Roskilde, he took up the study of excavated human bones more or less as a Sunday hobby. His hobby grew over the years until the point where he was recognized as a distinguished osteo-archaeologist: an expert in old bones and what they were able to show about the lives, aches and pains of their former owners.

In 1935 he began to collaborate with the Danish National Museum in the excavation of the large Abbey of the Augustinian Canons at Aebelholt in North Zealand, whose extensive burial grounds had remained in use from about 1175 until 1548. Møller-Christensen studied each skeleton as it was unearthed and, wherever the bones were reasonably well preserved, much information could be deduced about people of the Middle Ages and the diseases which once afflicted them. The undertaking represented an immense labour at the same time as it created access to an unrivalled collection of medieval anatomical material. The work would, in fact, take more than thirty years to complete, and not until 1968, after over a thousand bodies had been exhumed, was Møller-Christensen able to bring the Aebelholt project to a satisfactory conclusion.

The cast of the king's skull, which he now confronted, owed its presence in the pathological museum to a series of events that began on Tuesday, 17 February 1818. On that day the Rev. Peter Chalmers, minister of the abbey church, met with the heritors and magistrates in the Town House, Dunfermline, to discuss with William Burn, an architect from Edinburgh, plans for rebuilding the choir of Dunfermline Abbey. Their meeting was interrupted by the arrival of a workman from the abbey grounds, where work was already under way on clearing the site in the Psalter churchyard. While removing the top layers of earth, he told them, the men had found themselves exposing a great tomb, maybe the tomb of a royal person. In a flutter of excitement the meeting promptly adjourned to the churchyard.

All that could be seen of the tomb were two slabs of stone set flat in the ground: a larger stone that might cover a body and a smaller stone that might cover the head. From their position Mr Burn was able to comment that the stones lay in the very centre-line of the long-since demolished choir of the old abbey, immediately in front of where the high altar once stood. The larger stone, formerly a smooth broad table of gritty sandstone, six feet long and two feet four inches wide, seemed to have been fractured and broken by some immense force, perhaps by a falling mass of masonry. Embedded in its surface at regular intervals were three pairs of iron rings or handles, so decayed that some were loosened in their stone sockets. In line with this monumental slab and serving virtually as a headstone to the sepulchre, the smaller piece of sandstone was of similar width but a mere eighteen inches long. It had survived intact.

The slabs, when carefully moved aside, revealed a shallow vault barely eighteen inches deep, the walls lined with smooth-faced blocks of the same soft sandstone. The antiquarian eye of the Rev. Peter Chalmers noted how each stone bore the traditional mark of the master mason who originally worked on the tomb, but here, too, the stones were damaged, for a fissure over two inches wide split the vault from end to end. Recessed into the floor and only slightly smaller in its dimensions was yet another vault, lined with the same polished stone. Within the tomb, however, were no concealing slabs. The inner vault lay as an open grave. There had once been a coffin and a shroud, for what appeared to be fragments of oak, iron nails and shreds of cloth of gold were mouldering in the general debris.

Yet it was the tomb's occupant who dominated the scene, striking a momentary silence into the onlookers. The inner vault was almost completely taken up by the outline of a long figure, its entire body, head and limbs wrapped in a covering of dull lead. The encasings in fact consisted of two thin layers, each about an eighth of an inch thick. In some places they were corroded, gaps in the folds of lead at the breast, over one of the knees and around the toes making it possible to glimpse bare brown bones, evidently almost perfectly preserved. The opening of the tomb may have disturbed its contents, for some observers thought they could make out a rude crown about the figure's head, but others, hearing the whispers, were unable to spot it in the tomb's shadows.

Overawed no doubt by the sudden presence of the dead being, desecrated now, but almost certainly royal, the company faltered in its proceedings and came to a halt. A hasty graveside consultation recalled the legal obligations of the heritors and magistrates as trustees and guardians, the outcome being that Mr Burn undertook to set a workman to stand guard over the tomb until the proper authorities could be informed.

Dunfermline Abbey and its grounds came directly under the king's patronage, though it was administered in practice by a court composed of judges known as the Barons of the Exchequer. A message was therefore dispatched to Henry Jardine Esq., who bore the title of His Majesty's Remembrancer in the Exchequer and who almost by return sent back the order that, until the matter could be properly considered, the tomb should be resealed and made secure from further prying. Large stones were to be laid to replace those removed, and the sheriff was expressly charged with protecting the tomb from all 'mischievous depredation and idle intrusive curiosity'. The silent, waiting figure of the inner vault was thus once more shut off from light of day, this time beneath three great flagstones tightly bonded by iron bars.

That the occupant of the tomb was distinguished lay beyond dispute. The identity remained another question. The abbey walls were thought to shelter the burial places of at least nine kings, five queens, six princes and two princesses. Yet all at once the question became a matter of overwhelming interest far beyond the confines of Dunfermline, a widespread curiosity hinging on one point. Might this indeed be the body of King Robert the Bruce?

The exploits of the Bruce are probably more extensively and reliably documented than those of most ancient heroes who achieve a status of national legend, yet the story of this Scottish patriot still posed at least two unsolved historical puzzles. The first concerned his remains. What had become of his body? In the course of a turbulent history the Scots had somehow mislaid his tomb. The second concerned how he died. What finally brought down so great a hero? In the few surviving accounts of his death there is just the faint but intriguing suggestion of a medieval cover-up.

Time has done little to diminish the stature of Robert the Bruce. Six centuries after his death any sober assessment of his achievements still induces a reluctant admiration, even in Englishmen. Rebel, warrior, statesman and king, for over twenty years he inspired and led a bitter Scottish war of independence. Armed with little more than a sword and an indomitable resolution, he succeeded not only in wresting Scotland from the overlordship of the Plantagenet kings of England, but also, by winning the allegiance of warring factions within his own country, in masterminding the rebirth of Scotland as a united sovereign nation.

At the treaty of Northampton in 1328, England relinquished its claims upon Scotland, it being agreed that Scotland should 'according to its ancient boundaries in the days of Alexander IV . . . remain to Robert, King of Scots, his heirs and successors, free and divided from the Kingdom of England, without any subjection, right of service, claim or demands'. Bruce had won independence for his country and an undying reputation for himself. But even in his moment of greatest triumph the king was a doomed man, living out the final days of a personal tragedy. A little over a year after the treaty of Northampton he would be dead. For a long time now his physical strength had been slipping away under the onslaught of a slow, incurable illness and, fully aware of the disease's ravages and that he must die soon, he had shut himself away more and more from the world, delegating battles and conflicts to his lieutenants.

He in fact died at the age of fifty-five on 7 June 1329, but not even death could end his adventures. By a last wish he sought to fulfil an earlier vow to make, once peace and freedom had been restored to his kingdom, an expedition to the Holy Land and trounce the enemies of Christendom. His heart was to be removed from his body after death and transported to Jerusalem to be buried in the Church of the Holy Sepulchre, another Scottish hero, Sir James Douglas, being pledged to carry out this task. The heart was duly removed, embalmed and locked in a silver casket, which was then hung on a silver chain around Sir James's neck. The good knight set out with a considerable retinue, but as luck would have it his party found itself caught up in a local war in Spain in which it came to grief. In the end, Sir James Douglas's body and the silver casket were brought back to Scotland, the Bruce's heart being interred at last in Melrose Abbey. The historical records were not clear, however, over what became of the body after the heart had been taken out.

The Bruce certainly intended that he should be buried at Dunfermline Abbey. As the Chartulary of Dunfermline records: 'He chose his own interment to be among the kings of Scotland in the honourable monastery of Dunfermline.' His queen, who had died a year before him, was already interred there. A tomb was certainly prepared for him since, a year or so before his death, sculptors in Paris were ordered to prepare a monument of black marble, which, when set up in Dunfermline, was housed in a chapel of Baltic timber. The monument itself was brought to Dunfermline by way of Bruges, and great quantities of gold were purchased in Newcastle and York for its gilding.

By the end of the thirteenth century, Dunfermline Abbey was one of the most magnificently endowed establishments in Scotland and had replaced Iona as the recognized burial place for the Scottish kings. The weight of history was to rest so heavily on its walls, however, that it would go through the process of more than one rebuilding. The wars with the English took their toll, but in 1560 it was the Scots reformers who fell on the abbey with iconoclastic zeal. Their puritan enthusiasms led them to tear out and destroy every monument, image or relic, so stripping the interior down to a bare austerity. They wrecked the choir and transepts and left only the fabric of the nave intact, demoting this to the status of an ordinary parish church. In all the centuries' turmoils the great tomb of Robert the Bruce vanished without trace.

Clues to where it might lie existed in the writings of the monastic chroniclers. John of Fordun said the king had been interred 'in the middle of the choir with due honour'; and 'magnificently interred under the grand altar at Dunfermline Abbey'. The vast national epic poem, *The Brus* (1375), by John Barbour, Archdeacon of Aberdeen, though written over forty years after the Bruce's death, is usually accepted as being notably accurate in historical detail. This also specifies 'a fayr tumb, intill the Quer' as the burial place. The centre of the choir immediately before the high altar was therefore where any seeker might most expect to find it; and this was more or less the location of the tomb which the workmen unearthed in 1818.

Excitement grew that here indeed was the burial place of Scotland's national hero, and the Court of the Exchequer duly announced that it would give permission for the tomb to be reopened, but not until the walls of the new choir were completed and roofed over 'sufficiently to protect its contents and to exclude a crowd'. The tomb was then to be investigated with 'the assistance of gentlemen of science and knowledge of such subjects'.

Considering the intention to exclude a crowd, and presumably onlookers who were merely idle, vulgar or curious, it must have been a remarkably large party which arrived at the

Abbey Church on the morning of Friday, 5 November 1819, to witness the further probing of the tomb. The Court of the Exchequer was represented by the Lord Chief Baron as well as Mr Baron Clerk Rattray and His Majesty's Remembrancer in the Exchequer, Mr (later Sir) Henry Jardine. All the magistrates attended, as well as the Rev. Peter Chalmers, various parochial ministers and the heritors of the abbey. Three doctors were present: Dr Gregory, His Majesty's first physician in Scotland, Dr Munro, Professor of Anatomy at the University of Edinburgh, and Robert Liston, destined to become one of the most famous surgeons of his day. The party was completed by Mr Burn, the architect, various other men of science, a considerable number of gentlemen of the county and the principal citizens of Dunfermline. The main party was not to be admitted until 11 a.m., but the day began at nine when Mr Jardine arrived with Mr Burn. The three bonded flagstones were then removed and a deep trench, three feet wide, dug entirely round the original vault.

As soon as the tomb was open and the vanguard party admitted, it could be seen at once that a rapid deterioration had occurred since the original discovery. The gold cloth had suffered badly. It was now reduced to fragments a few inches in size, and even these tended to moulder into dust when touched. Scraps of the shroud were, however, carefully collected and preserved, sealed between sheets of glass. In the bottom of the inner vault a deposit of black dust now lay two or three inches deep. Henry Jardine carefully sifted through the layer, paying particular attention to the areas below the hands. He hoped to turn up any rings that might have fallen from the fingers, but found only decayed pieces of coffin oak and two or three iron nails with very broad heads.

After the south side of the vault had been dismantled, a wooden eighteen-inch board with a sharpened edge was slipped under the body and the whole carefully raised to rest on the rim of the vault. Measurements showed the remains to be those of a man five feet eleven inches or even six feet tall, but the full extent of the deterioration at last grew clear. The enfolding lead coverings were now corroded and broken in many places. The breast bone, visible through one of the defects in the lead and in its normal position when the vault was first opened, had since collapsed. Henry Jardine also noted the absence of the rude crown which had been spoken about and quietly assumed it must have been purloined at the previous disinterment.

The lead could be folded back from the body and limbs, but the casing was so firm and solid about the head that a saw was needed to expose the skull. Eventually the skeleton was completely in view, and, apart from a few traces where the larynx had been, every sign of softer tissue, even the various ligaments and cartilages, had disappeared. Only the bones remained. Each bone could be lifted out of position without disturbing any other, even the individual vertebral bones of the spine. Yet despite the fact that its bones had collapsed, the chest was the most startling feature. The breast bone had most certainly been carefully split along its length as though to allow for the heart's removal.

Dr Gregory could restrain his sense of theatre no longer. He clambered down into the freshly dug trench, grasped the skull and held it triumphantly aloft. 'This', he announced to the crowding onlookers, 'is the head of King Robert!'

The skull which Dr Gregory displayed retained, even in its gaunt skeletal features, an impression of strength, of high flaring cheekbones, of a square, heavy-jawed determination. In spite of the dampness it seemed almost perfectly preserved. A considerable quantity of water ran out when Henry Jardine, in a moment of curiosity, inserted a finger into the large aperture at the base of the skull which gives entrance to the cranial cavity. In the lower jaw the teeth survived, but in the centre of the upper jaw, one group of front teeth, the incisors, was missing. The bone of the upper jaw which should have contained the sockets for these teeth was itself curiously eroded. The doctors agreed the distortion must have occurred during life, and Liston suggested a fracture from a battle wound, an idea embraced with enthusiasm.

Dr Munro had had the foresight to bring with him from Edinburgh a young artist so that a pictorial record might be kept of any objects of importance discovered during the exhumation. The artist, Mr Scoular, was a pupil of the sculptor Sir Francis Chantrey, and it was to Mr Scoular's care that the skull would be temporarily entrusted. In the meantime, a meticulous examination of the rest of the skeleton showed little else to discover, and so the body's components were carefully put back together. Then the doors at the north and south ends of the new choir were thrown open to the immense crowd gathered in the churchyard, who filed slowly and respectfully past their dead monarch whose identity was established by strong circumstantial evidence if not by ultimate proof.

All had not been so respectful behind the closed doors, however, as Dr Gregory discovered when he tarried at the Queensferry Inn on his return to Edinburgh. One of the doctors accompanying him gleefully produced a small bone from the foot of the skeleton, having abstracted it as a souvenir. Dr Gregory discreetly settled for preserving the bone in a small bottle and labelling it carefully.

In the days which followed, workmen dismantled the old vault and prepared a new one. While clearing the debris and rubble around the old tomb, they discovered a sealed lead casket about eleven feet from the north-east corner of the vault. The casket contained lime and what appeared to be preserved animal tissues which were probably the embalmed internal organs and intestines from a royal burial. Although Barbour's *The Brus* described the king as having been disembowelled cleanly and embalmed richly, the distance of the casket from the grave made it impossible to be certain whether the two were connected.

A few days later, on 10 November, the workmen made yet another discovery. This time it was a small, rough, copper coffin-plate, bearing the inscription *Robertus Scotorum Rex*. It was immediately accepted as incontrovertible proof of identity, and only some years later did the truth leak out. It had in fact been placed as a hoax skilfully perpetrated by three high-spirited young men, their ringleader being the younger brother of the architect William Burn.

In due course the king was reinterred, his bones carefully replaced in their lead wrappings and laid within a large lead coffin. Small lead caskets containing coins and various biographies, including Barbour's epic poem, were placed beside him, and at Dr Gregory's instigation the whole collection was sealed by filling the coffin with melted pitch. There were to be no further intrusions. The coffin was then placed in the new vault, beneath the very centre of the rebuilt choir at the exact spot where it had been discovered. As a mark of nineteenth-century respect, Mr Burn altered the design for the tower of the new choir to frame the four words KING ROBERT THE BRUCE within its parapets.

Robert Liston, the surgeon, prepared a short statement on the anatomical features of the skull. Dr Gregory wrote a long facetious account of the episode in a letter to a friend. Henry Jardine's report of the proceedings was considered not only by the Barons of the Exchequer but also by the Society of Antiquaries of Scotland; and even the Rev. Peter Chalmers felt compelled to write an account in a book published more than twenty years later. The work of Mr Scoular, the young artist, was, however, the most important contribution. From the skull he prepared not a drawing but a single, superb cast, an exact replica of the original skull that Dr Gregory had flourished above the grave. This original cast, mounted and varnished, remains a treasured possession of the Anatomical Museum of the Medical School of the University of Edinburgh. One copy of the cast was deposited in the Museum of the Royal College of Surgeons of England in London, and another was placed in a protective glass case to be reverently displayed in the new choir of the Abbey Church of Dunfermline.

The king's mortal remains were safe from further attention, but the existence of the cast of the skull raised the intriguing possibility that it might hold a clue to the puzzle of which illness brought down an illustrious monarch. Any historical view of his disease depended very much on partisan attitudes. The English chronicles tended to state bluntly that he died a leper, and the French chronicler, Jean Le Bel, wrote in 1327 that the king was a victim of *la grosse maladie*, a term usually taken to signify leprosy. On the other hand, no single contemporary Scottish source said it was leprosy from which the king suffered, while surviving descriptions of his malady are diagnostically far from clear.

Leprosy is a notoriously feared disease in the context of recorded history. Descriptions of it can be recognized in ancient Egyptian, Indian and Chinese as well as biblical writings, and, while skeletal evidence is largely lacking from before the Christian era, an anthropomorphic jar, dated to about 1400 BC and discovered in Jordan, may well show a leprous individual. The troops of the Roman Empire are said to have carried the disease to Spain. In medieval times, the journeyings of the Crusaders are thought to have been a primary aid in its spread, since the great, slow wave of a leprosy epidemic reached its zenith in Northern and Western Europe during the thirteenth century before gradually beginning to recede. In a few places, including Scandinavia, pockets of infection lingered on into the late nineteenth century.

Modern science knows leprosy as a chronic, infectious disease which is caused by the bacillus *Mycobacterium leprae*. This concentrates its long-term onslaught on the skin, the mucous membrane linings of the nose, throat and mouth, and the body's peripheral nerves. To the medieval mind, by contrast, it was an infliction visited on its victims as a sign of divine disapproval for some moral failing, especially for wanton or lustful living. Even today the term 'social leper' carries with it uncharitable undertones of moral judgement.

With his warning bell or clapper and his traditional cry of 'Unclean!', the haunting figure of the leper was fated to walk through history enduring not only the distressing disfigurements of his illness but also the rejection of whatever society he happened to live in. He was a pitiful object of moral as well as of physical revulsion, and the medieval church went so far as to make provision for a special service to be performed 'for the seclusion of a leper' which was virtually a counterpart to the burial of the dead.

The sufferer was to be dressed in identifiable dark clothing, then brought to church. On entering the building he was to make his last confession. A black cloth was spread on trestles before the altar and the sufferer knelt beneath it. After hearing mass, he was led through the presbytery to a quiet place where the priest cast a symbolic spadeful of earth upon each foot, saying: 'Be thou dead to the world, but alive again in

God.' Ten special rules were next read out to him so that he might 'live on earth in peace with his neighbours', and the Ten Commandments were finally recited, 'so that he might live in heaven with the saints'. Until that time came he was to be considered an outcast among men.

In fact the prohibitions must have effectively prevented any association with neighbours. The leper had always to wear his special clothing so that he might be recognized. He was forbidden to enter churches, markets, mills, bakehouses, shops, taverns or houses, or any assembly of people. He was not allowed to eat or drink in any company except that of other lepers. When he went out he was not to answer anyone who spoke to him until he had stepped from the path and stood to leeward of them, and he was to enter no narrow lanes or passageways in case he should meet a person face to face. The prohibition extended even beyond death. He was not to be buried within a churchyard unless special dispensation was granted.

The leper was then assigned a hut in an isolated location where he must go to live out his life, and in time such groups of huts developed into leper communities and eventually, as the need for care and attention became more clearly recognized, into more permanent buildings: the leper hospitals of medieval Europe. It is possible that there were about 19,000 leprosariums in Europe by the time Robert the Bruce was born, and leper houses had certainly been established in both Edinburgh and Glasgow by the early fourteenth century.

We are familiar today with the clinical descriptions of leprosy. It is, in fact, only a moderately infectious disease, and prolonged and close contact, as in family groups, is needed to pass it from person to person. Its onset is, however, slow and insidious, and it may be present for years before even the early symptoms become detectable. A rather ill-defined rash on the body, some nasal congestion, perhaps even an inflamed eye – these symptoms could all have other causes. The real tell-tale sign emerges when any areas of skin become anaesthetized to touch or sensation. This represents the first clinical evidence of damage to peripheral nerves.

How ruthlessly the disease progresses depends a good deal on an individual patient's resistance to the bacilli. Where there is little resistance, the illness's slow advance will lead to a thickening and drying of the skin, particularly on the face, with a corrugating of the skin's folds and the formation of nodules. All facial hair, including eyebrows and eyelashes, eventually disappears. The nasal cartilage and palate may be attacked and destroyed, and the face then takes on the classic leonine appearance of the leper. Serious burns become a constant hazard because of the loss of sensation in the nerves. Muscles grow weak, and in the end there may also be gross deformations of the hands and feet.

It is thought that leprosy died out in the temperate areas of Europe as a consequence of better standards of living and the greater consciousness of hygiene which these brought with them. This has defined it today as a Third World disease, widespread in subtropical and tropical regions from Central and South America to Africa, the Near East and large tracts of Asia. Since the 1940s slow-acting drugs have been available which can halt the disease's progress or even achieve a cure. Nevertheless there are said to be as many as ten million lepers in the world at the present time. Leprosy is second only to tuberculosis as a major cause of chronic disability among humankind.

Whether the disease which is called leprosy today is precisely the same as the disease known by that name in the Middle Ages has been a rich area for academic debate. A disease can change its character fundamentally over the

course of 700 years, even over the course of a single generation. Scarlet fever is a case in point. Within living memory it
was a scourge fully capable of wiping out all the young
children in a family within a week, yet it has evolved to
become the relatively innocuous disease which does little
more than cause some unpleasant discomfort and maybe
disrupt a child's school work or holiday. So far as leprosy is
concerned, the further we go back into history the harder
precise diagnostic details become to verify. It was this fact
which màde the work of Dr Møller-Christensen among his
medieval skeletons so valuable.

In 1944, while working at Aebelholt Abbey, he had
unearthed the skeleton of a young woman, aged between
twenty-five and thirty, who must have died in about 1250.
Her bones showed remarkable signs of deformity and disease.
Møller-Christensen was perplexed; he had seen nothing like
it before. He took the skeleton to both Copenhagen and Oslo,
but the authorities he consulted were equally mystified; the
pathological museums there contained nothing resembling
this disorder. At last he offered a tentative diagnosis: perhaps
it was a case of leprosy. He was no expert in leprosy, but it
seemed to him that any disorder which damaged the bones
so drastically yet spared the skull might just possibly be
leprosy. He was aware that modern leprosy did not produce
the bone changes he had found, but leprosy, as we have said,
could have changed its character since medieval times.

The only way of testing his hypothesis would be by
comparing the skeleton to those of known medieval lepers,
and at this point he made a surprising discovery. Despite the
broad spread of leprosy in the thirteenth century, nowhere
did there exist a collection to demonstrate the bone changes
of leprosy from medieval times onward. If he was to make a
comparison with reference to a museum of the pathological

changes of leprosy, then he was going to have to form the collection himself.

This formidable prospect seems to have left him undaunted. In medieval Denmark, leper hospitals were usually dedicated to St George (St Jørgen), and Denmark, he discovered, had possessed at least thirty-one St Jørgen hospitals, each with its own burial ground. There was therefore a chance that one such burial ground might prove accessible to excavation. It would be safe to assume that practically every person interred within that burial ground could be regarded as a victim of leprosy, and thus his plan, quite simply, was to establish a collection by excavating bodies from the burial ground of a known leper colony.

In practice the idea did not turn out to be so easily realized. Many leper burial grounds had been brought into general use after their St Jørgen's hospital had been abandoned. Others had disappeared beneath the streets and buildings of expanding towns. Then Møller-Christensen recalled a moment from his early days as a doctor, after he had just qualified and was working as a medical assistant at the hospital in Naestved, a town about fifty miles south-west of Copenhagen. One day he accompanied his chief on a trip to visit a patient. They had taken a route that ran along the Suså, the main waterway of Naestved, and here his chief had paused to point out a meadow which lay on the bank of the stream. 'This is the spot', he informed him, 'where the St Jørgen hospital of Naestved is supposed to have stood.'

The Sunday after the memory returned, Møller-Christensen placed a spade in the boot of his car and drove to Naestved. He was baffled to find the place almost unrecognizable; the meadow had vanished beneath a factory. Unwilling to abandon his quest so easily, Møller-Christensen paused to question people who lived in surrounding properties. They were all very definite. They had watched the factory being built, but certainly no skeletons had been unearthed when its foundations were dug. Was it possible that his old chief could have been slightly off target with the spot he had indicated? Møller-Christensen began the task of calling on every family in the vicinity of the factory, asking whether any of them had ever unearthed any human bones in their gardens. 'In most places,' he wrote later, 'the good people took my question for a silly idea engendered by the heat and accompanied me to the door with a pitying smile.' At last his dogged single-mindedness was rewarded. He was told of a farmer who had found some human skulls in his yard when laying a deep sewer fifteen years before. The farm lay about 200 metres from the factory and was known as St Jørgen's Farm.

The farmer met the doctor's excited approaches with courtesy and kindness. He was indeed able to confirm that they had dug up human skulls when laying the deep sewer. In fact, many human bones had been discovered about the farm. It was his opinion that the farm must have been built over the site of an old warrior grave. Yet so convincing and infectious was Møller-Christensen's enthusiasm that the farmer invited him to test his theory then and there. Thus, on that hot Sunday afternoon in August 1948, Dr Møller-Christensen took off his jacket and began to dig a large hole in the middle of the farmyard only a few feet from the farmer's back door. Within a few hours he had exposed an untouched grave and a set of human bones which showed the unmistakable deformities of the hands and feet of a leper.

Dr Møller-Christensen's powers of persuasion must have been remarkable. The farmer agreed to allow a gradual and prolonged excavation of his property, though he can have had little idea of the implications at the outset. His farmhouse and outbuildings turned out to be built on top of the old graveyard.

Preliminary digging showed up the foundations of a small gothic church directly under the archway which gave the only access to the farm's courtyard. The Naestved Museum, hearing of the project, undertook to excavate the masonry foundations and to reconstruct a ground plan of the original church and its burial ground. Meanwhile every spadeful of soil turned over in the yard seemed to reveal one more grave and yet another beautifully preserved skeleton. And Dr Møller-Christensen, it became certain, would not be content with exhuming just a sample of skeletons. He was clearly not going to rest until he had dug up the entire churchyard.

The exhumation of certain bodies proved impossible for the time being, since they were in places partly overlain by the farmhouse walls. This problem was eventually resolved in 1966 when the town of Naestved bought St Jørgen's Farm and demolished the buildings. By July 1968 the site had been totally excavated. During a project that caught him up in twenty years of work, Dr Møller-Christensen unearthed, examined, cleaned, preserved and stored more than 650 skeletons.

Alongside the years of excavation had gone an investigation into the bone changes which might occur in leprosy, though it was unlikely that much would emerge which could help with any analysis of the mystery of Robert the Bruce's illness. The king's skeleton itself was secured to await eternity in its matrix of pitch. So far as was known no effects of leprosy had ever shown up on the bones of any victim's skull, and only the plaster skull remained available for examination. Discussion about the king's illness had been able to proceed only for the most part on a basis of studying the conflicting and imprecise historical records. The earliest mention of any illness came in a letter written in July 1327, during a visit to Ulster where the Bruce forced a truce on Sir Henry

Mandeville, the Seneschal. The writer, a hostile eyewitness, declared that the king had leprosy and was so feeble and struck down by illness that he could not live till the following August, 'for he can scarcely move anything but his tongue'. The king was present at the Edinburgh Parliament in March 1328, although confined to bed. By July he was too weak to attend the marriage of his son, an important political match which was to seal the peace with England. In the early months of 1329, he was carried on a slow and painful pilgrimage to Whithorn in Galloway to seek the intercession of St Ninian in his illness, but then he returned home to die in June of the same year.

King Robert's last years were mostly passed in quiet seclusion. He had built a home for himself at Cardross, on the north shore of the Firth of Clyde. His time was spent in improving the grounds, in his favourite sport of hawking, in sailing and in involving himself in the art of shipbuilding. He had kept a fool to entertain him and a lion as a pet, and there was no evidence whatsoever of any attempt to segregate him from his family or friends. Even courtiers or foreign diplomats could freely gain admission for an audience. What the king or his physicians thought his illness could have been is not recorded in any account. Barbour's epic poem *The Brus* refers to a severe, chronic illness caused by the hardships which the king suffered during his earlier years, 'lying cold' upon the ground. In the same poem the Bruce is depicted as accepting his illness as a punishment for his misdeeds:

> 'For through my strife I bear the guilt
> Of blood that has been freely spilt,
> And harmless men that have been slain,
> Therefore this illness and this pain,
> My recompense I take to be.'

The main arguments against accepting the claims of the English and French chroniclers have centred on the question of precisely what was meant by the term leprosy in the thirteenth and fourteenth centuries, especially since it seems likely that other clinical conditions were sometimes confused with it. Any skin condition which caused gross disfigurement, even psoriasis, may have been mistakenly labelled as leprosy; and while some early writings on leprosy speak of an issue or discharge, such phrases fit more readily into a description of severe, untreated venereal disease.

In 1924, the scientist Karl Pearson did in fact offer this alternative suggestion. Could it have been that Robert the Bruce was suffering from syphilis? Even in modern times, syphilis and leprosy have occasionally been mistaken for one another. Robert the Bruce was in many ways a traditional monarch of his times. His private life had been conducted with the same ruthless energy as his public one. There had been many mistresses and he had acknowledged several illegitimate children. Warnings of various plots against him were said to have been whispered into his ear by lady friends in intimate, secluded moments.

> And many times, as I heard say,
> Through women that he with would play,
> That would tell him all that they might hear,

wrote John Barbour, Archdeacon of Aberdeen.

Karl Pearson suggested it was just possible to make out small pits in the surface of Scoular's cast, and a pitting of the cranial bones of the skull would certainly have tended to support his diagnosis. The appearance had been accentuated, on the other hand, by small pockets of dust which had gradually accumulated, and he admitted that all the marks he observed could have come from flaws in the casting process or even from wear and minor damage to the cast itself. The most formidable obstacle to his theory, however, lay in the fact that Robert the Bruce had died over a century and a half before the generally accepted date for the first appearance of syphilis in Western Europe. Syphilis has traditionally been regarded as a disease of the New World, for it seems to have swept across Europe in an explosive pandemic towards the end of the fifteenth century, conventional belief associating its appearance with the return of Columbus's crew after their discovery of America in 1492.

The medical profession noted Karl Pearson's suggestion with interest, but regarded it as unproven. It seemed highly improbable that Robert the Bruce could have been a rare, sporadic case of syphilis without starting his own epidemic. The controversy continued on its way, some authorities insisting that a diagnosis of leprosy was untenable, others doubting whether it would ever be possible to make any diagnosis at all. Scoular's cast was destined to remain on the shelf in the anatomical museum as an intriguing puzzle for 146 years.

Møller-Christensen's excavations at St Jørgen's Farm had, on the other hand, begun to bear fruit with the very first skeletons exposed, since these displayed evidence of bone changes never before described in leprosy. As his work proceeded and the pathological collection was assembled, the bone changes came to be established beyond all question. In nearly three quarters of the collection there were small but characteristic changes in the bones of the upper jaw and nasal region, the bones of the upper jaw having been eroded and worn away in the area of the central teeth. The upper incisor teeth had thus become loosened in their sockets and in many cases were missing. The small spine of bone which supports the cartilaginous tissues of the nose seemed to have atrophied and withered. This group of changes in the skull Dr Møller-Christensen christened *facies leprosa*.

While leprosy had long been known to cause infiltration and chronic inflammation of the tissues about the nose and mouth, no one had hitherto suspected that the bones of the nose and upper jaw might also be damaged. The questions now posed were, first, was this a characteristic of medieval leprosy, and second, had the behaviour of the disease subsequently changed? X-ray studies began at once on modern leprosy cases, and, armed with a knowledge of what they were looking for, investigators found the search easy. *Facies leprosa* was present in between half and three quarters of samples of cases in Norway, the Belgian Congo and India. Further studies showed that the bone changes occurred quite early in the disease process. To Dr Møller-Christensen's delight, his archaeological delvings had added new knowledge to the understanding of leprosy. His contribution also made it somewhat easier for a doctor to detect and confirm the presence of leprosy in its early stages. Early diagnosis meant early treatment; early treatment meant early arrest of the disease process. Møller-Christensen's work has been called by Calvin Wells 'an admirable example of how the story of an ancient disease has helped diagnosis in living patients'.

Møller-Christensen had thrown an entirely fresh beam of light on to the pathology of leprosy. His researches had also shown how the natural history of leprosy remained completely unchanged over the centuries, medieval leprosy and modern leprosy being identical in their effect. Only one irony remained. The young woman from Aebelholt whose skeleton had set him in the way of his quest was shown beyond dispute by the pathological collection never to have had leprosy. Her disease remained undiagnosed.

The years of research had established Møller-Christensen as a scientist with an international reputation. His days as a general practitioner were left far behind. He had been appointed Professor of the History of Medicine at the University of Copenhagen, and a museum had been set up to store and display his pathological collections. In the midst of his academic duties, he continued with excavations, with delivering lectures to societies and learned associations, with the preparation of articles and books, with journeys abroad to study leprosy and other pathological collections and archaeological material. In Denmark, he was regarded with affectionate wonder and respect; abroad, he became something of a legend.

In Graham Greene's novel *A Burnt-out Case*, Dr Colin, a doctor who has given his life to working in a leper colony in Africa, describes an almost mythical figure unconsciously touched by divine mission:

There is an old Danish doctor still going the rounds who became a leprologist late in life. By accident. He was excavating an ancient cemetery and found skeletons there without finger-bones – it was an old leper-cemetery of the fourteenth century. He X-rayed the skeletons and he made discoveries in the bones, especially in the nasal area, which were quite unknown to any of us . . . You will meet him at any international conference on leprosy carrying his skull with him in an airline's overnight bag. It has passed through a lot of *douaniers'* hands. It must be rather a shock, that skull, to them, but I believe they don't charge duty on it.

The pen portrait seems clearly based on the real-life original of Professor Møller-Christensen. In 1963, he went to Paris for a week to look for evidence of *facies leprosa* in the skulls of the catacombs. His companion, Dr W. H. Joppling, was startled and amused by the unconcerned way he walked through the streets, carrying skulls like vegetables in a string bag and oblivious to the sidelong glances of passers-by.

In 1968, Møller-Christensen made his trip to Edinburgh. He was there able to study the skull and skeletons preserved in the anatomical museum of the university, and was as a matter of course shown Scoular's cast of the skull of Robert the Bruce. Without hesitation he diagnosed *facies leprosa*. The eroded upper jaw and missing teeth, which the surgeon Robert Liston had once attributed to a fracture sustained in battle, were the unequivocal marks of leprosy. To back his case the professor could produce a whole museum of skulls for comparison. The matter finally lay beyond dispute. A great man had been brought low by a terrible affliction. Robert the Bruce, King of Scots and hero of his country, ended his days as a leper.

Chapter 12

The Walk to Eternity

The Far-Eastern Sledge Party, a small team of three men with seventeen sledge dogs and three sledges, left base camp on Commonwealth Bay at thirty minutes past noon on Sunday, 10 November 1912, and climbed slowly eastward across long ice-slopes through a calm sunny afternoon. It was one arm only of the Australasian Antarctic Expedition of 1911–14, but an important one, since Douglas Mawson, the expedition's leader, headed the party himself.

Mawson was just thirty years old: tall and lean with fair hair, a long thin face, a high forehead and a perpetually solemn expression. He was a scientist, a geologist of the first rank, already widely respected for his field studies in remote regions hitherto unexplored. The expedition he led was superbly organized and equipped. The Australian party was the first polar expedition to maintain radio contact with the outside world, for Mawson paused on the outward voyage to set up a wireless relay station at Macquarie Island in the Southern Ocean. He had earlier declined an invitation to join Scott's expedition to the South Pole, which set out in October the previous year and from whom nothing had yet been heard.

Operating under the auspices of the Australian Government, Mawson's expedition undertook to explore the part of the Antarctic continent and coastline which lay closest to

Australia. It was planned as a three-pronged assault. The expedition ship, the *Aurora*, had landed the two widely separated Eastern and Western Shore Parties before sailing along the coast, charting and exploring as much of the huge stretch of coastline between the parties as the ice allowed the vessel to reach. The two shore parties then spent the Antarctic winter sheltering in respective base camps, waiting for the improved conditions of the short summer before fanning out in a series of cross-country marches to survey as much as possible of the hinterland. At the earliest opportunity, the various teams embarked on their summer activities with pent-up energy.

In organizing his programme of research and exploration, Mawson could draw on plenty of personal experience. He was already a seasoned Antarctic explorer, having spent two years as a member of Shackleton's 1907 'Farthest South' expedition when he was with the first party to climb to the summit of Mount Erebus, the 13,370-foot-high, active volcano that stands on the shores of the Ross Sea. He had taken measurements of its crater, and as physicist to the party accomplished vast quantities of work in geomagnetic and auroral studies, besides carrying out precise triangulation surveys. While Shackleton was on his great southern march, Mawson had been a member of a three-man sledge team that made a round trek of 1,250 miles to locate the ever-changing position of the South Magnetic Pole.

Now he divided his Eastern Shore Party into six sledge teams, each consisting of three men. To each team he assigned a definite objective. The first team, with the second team in support, was to strike directly inland to locate yet again the varying position of the South Magnetic Pole and make geomagnetic observations. A third team was to explore the hinterland to the west, an area which could be surveyed from the sea. The three remaining teams were all to travel eastward, for here the sea was covered by mile after mile of solid ice, making any approach by ship impossible. He had tentatively divided this coastline into three adjoining regions, each between 100 and 150 miles long, allocating a region to each sledge team. The region most distant from base he reserved for himself. This Far-Eastern Sledge Party, as his team came to be known, faced the most arduous task, for it had furthest to go and carried the heaviest load of provisions.

To accompany him on the journey Mawson chose Xavier Mertz, a cheerful, irrepressible 28-year-old law graduate from Basle in Switzerland, who addressed his companions in idiosyncratic English, and Lieutenant Ninnis, a resolute but oddly formal 22-year-old lieutenant from the Royal Inniskilling Fusiliers. Ninnis had delighted his fellow explorers by embarking on shipboard accompanied by trunk after trunk of dress uniforms and highly polished boots. Mertz was the reigning World Champion Ski-runner, and both Ninnis and Mertz, from the moment they joined the expedition, laboured to make themselves expert at handling sledge dogs. All three men were trained to a peak of fitness.

As they moved off that Sunday afternoon, their three sledges, each between eleven and twelve feet long, cut deep tracks into the snow. They were carrying over three quarters of a ton of supplies and equipment. Indeed, so precise were Mawson's preparations that he knew the combined laden weight of the sledges to be 1,723 pounds 11·3 ounces. As provisions were consumed, the sledges were to be abandoned, and each man had been allowed only the barest minimum of personal effects. For Douglas Mawson, these were his diary and a photograph folded protectively inside his wallet. Before sailing he had managed to persuade Francisca Adriana Delprait, a girl he had nicknamed 'Paquita', to promise to marry him on his return from Antarctica. The photograph was her portrait.

The first afternoon was only a preliminary march. During the night they rested at Aladdin's Cave, an artificial cavern dug deep inside the ice about five miles from base where a cache of spare supplies was stored. Early next morning they started out beneath overcast skies upon the real journey. By midday, they were struggling through falling snow driven by 40 m.p.h. winds. By early afternoon, snow torn from the surface of the ice was being thrown up as drift, a thick grey-white haze that shrouded everything, and the wind was rising. They stopped and made camp, and soon their tent was half-buried, their sledges hidden by drift, the dogs visible only as small huddled mounds, curled against each other in the tent's leeside. For two days they lay listening to the canvas thrashing in the storm. By the third night, the gales had Mawson feeling so insecure that he thought it advisable to sleep with the more valuable equipment inside his sleeping-bag in case the tent gave way. By the end of the first week they had spent almost five days sheltering, pressing forward during brief intervals when the wind dropped and the drift cleared. Barely twenty-five miles had been covered, and they were thankful to meet up with one of the other Eastern Sledge Parties which was dropping off extra supplies for them.

Now the weather improved, but the terrain as they pressed eastwards kept progress frustratingly slow. In places they struggled for mile after mile across sastrugi, an ice-surface scoured by the wind into pitted corrugations which resembled nothing so much as sharp-edged frozen waves. Time after time they slipped, falling heavily as they tried to step or jump from crest to crest. It was a relief when they came to broad tracts of smooth snow where Mertz could don skis and travel ahead, though here the apparently firm crust might treacherously give way at any moment to reveal the firmly packed layer as only a few feet thick and bridging a seemingly bottomless crevasse.

They worked their way across frozen valleys, skirted sudden drops, discovered mounds by stumbling over them. For three days they marched towards a distant mountain whose peak seemed to beckon them to the unexplored territory on the other side. They called it Aurora Peak, after their ship, and beyond it could see the low sun caught and reflected in the far-away ice-cliffs of the first great glacier blocking their path. This they christened Mertz Glacier, and spent anxious days picking a way through the broken maze of crevasses which fissured its surface. A hundred miles further on they came to a second glacier, which they named after Ninnis, its surface crumpled into huge ice-waves with crests 250 feet high and over a mile apart.

On good days they made as many as seventeen or eighteen miles; on bad days they managed no more than four or five. When the weather broke they lay up for days on end, listening to 75 m.p.h. gales tearing at the canvas while suffering the agony of cramped conditions which did not even allow them room to stretch their limbs. During these periods of forced inactivity, they reduced rations and endured hunger-provoked vivid, disturbing dreams. At night Mawson would wake to hear Ninnis calling 'Hike! Hike!' to his dogs in his sleep. Sometimes they tried to read, for Ninnis had brought a single volume of Thackeray and Mertz a collection of Sherlock Holmes stories. Mertz's book, however, was finished too soon, and he passed the time trying to recount the stories to the others. Hardships were beginning to take their toll. Ninnis, after suffering a bout of snow-blindness, developed an abscess on a finger. When he could bear the increasing pain no longer, he begged Mawson to lance it. The act was done with a pocket knife. Mawson himself was suffering from a split and swollen lip which sent shafts of pain throbbing along the side of his head and face.

The dogs presented their own special problems. In the mornings it was sometimes necessary to free their frozen coats from the ice before they could move. A sick or injured animal was allowed to run along with the party unharnessed until it died or recovered, but they could carry no passengers. Any animal which became too weak to pull again was killed.

By 13 December they were over 300 miles from base camp. It was almost time to turn back. They had already abandoned one sledge. The next day was promisingly sunny with little cloud, light winds and a temperature rising to only 11° below freezing-point. They were able to make a rapid push across smooth snow-fields, Mertz singing student songs at the top of his voice as he led on skis. At midday they paused to take the regular noon observation of latitude, and then Mawson worked out their position as they travelled, riding on the first sledge. He was engrossed in his calculations when Mertz paused in his singing, held a ski-stick aloft and then went on. Here was their prearranged signal to indicate a crevasse. Mawson called back a warning to Ninnis, and for a quarter of a mile his sledge ran smoothly ahead. He interrupted his calculations only to speak absent-mindedly to the dogs as he heard a distant whimper from the following pack. All at once he realized that Mertz had stopped and was staring back in bewilderment. Mawson turned and found himself gazing on an empty landscape.

As Mawson leapt from his sledge and stumbled back along the tracks, he prayed that a rise in the ground had simply hidden Ninnis from view. The hope was still-born. Where

Mertz had paused to hold his ski-stick aloft there yawned a gaping hole. The lid of a crevasse had collapsed, leaving a crater over eleven feet across. The tracks of two sledges approached the gap; only one set left it. Testing the ground, Mawson crawled cautiously to the edge and peered down into a dark, ice-walled abyss. He called into the crevasse but heard only the reverberations of his own voice in the frozen stillness.

The gap was too wide to be bridged by a sledge. Together he and Mertz broke back the snow-crust to firm ground and then, secured by a rope, Mawson leaned out over the edge. Far below was a ledge, a small projecting shelf of ice with two dogs on it, one already dead, the other writhing with a broken back. There was the dark shape of the tent, one of the food packs; nothing else. Beneath the ledge the crevasse plummeted into engulfing blackness.

With knotted fishing lines they sounded the distance to the ledge: 150 feet of sheer ice wall. It was beyond the reach of all the ropes from the remaining sledge lashed together. For three hours they took turns to hang above the crevasse and call in case Ninnis was only stunned and had regained consciousness. It was an impotent gesture born from an inability to accept that he could be dead so suddenly. As they watched, the injured dog ceased its intermittent spasms and lay still.

At last, in numb withdrawal from the catastrophe, they climbed a few miles to the highest point in the landscape to establish their position and take stock. They were immediately south of Cape Freshfield, 315 miles from base camp, and their circumstances were perilous. There were no depots left behind them since they intended returning by an alternative route, and only that morning had Mawson reapportioned the loads on the two remaining sledges. One final incisive dash was to be made to the east, to reach the furthest point possible before heading for home. One sledge only was to be used in this forced march, a sledge pulled by the weaker and more exhausted animals and carrying supplies for just a few days. At the completion of the march, the sledge was to be abandoned, the other sledge, packed with the bulk of provisions, having been cached meanwhile and its dog team, the stronger, healthier huskies, rested in preparation for the long journey back.

In organizing his order of march, Mawson's logic had been realistic and direct. He reasoned that should a snow-bridge collapse, it would most likely do so beneath the first sledge to cross. He had therefore led with the sledge to be abandoned, leaving the one carrying the bulk of supplies to follow over tested ground. But it was the second sledge which had with Ninnis fallen to destruction. Mertz and Mawson were stranded seven weeks from base with little food, an exhausted dog team and only some ill-assorted remnants of equipment.

Together they returned to the crevasse and stripped down the remaining sledge, scrutinizing every item of its load. There was a spare tent canvas but no tent poles; sleeping-bags but no changes of clothing; ration packs enough for two for a little over a week and the cooker with some fuel, but no food whatsoever for the dogs. In discarding equipment they spared only written records, camera and films in a ruthless elimination of excess weight. Mawson, making a cool calculation, decided they just might get out alive – if they used the dogs as food as they went. With desperate economy they threw left-over rawhide straps and worn-out fur gloves for the dogs to gnaw on, boiling up old discarded food bags to brew a thin, watery soup for themselves.

Then, one last time, they called into the unanswering chasm. As they stood beside the crevasse, two tiny figures amid the eternal whiteness, Mawson, in awkward tones, read the funeral service aloud before at length, at 9 p.m., they forced themselves to turn and leave. In the perpetual twilight of an Antarctic summer evening they began their bid for survival. In his diary Mawson concluded a terse account of the tragedy and their predicament with a simple phrase: 'May God help us.'

For a while they travelled with blind disregard for danger, plunging recklessly down snow-covered slopes, scarcely bothering to plot a route. Mawson wrote of an almost languid acceptance that the next crevasse would be the last. In five and a half hours they were back to the campsite of the previous night where they had abandoned the third sledge. Mertz broke a runner from it and cut it in two. Lashed to the skis, the pieces provided a framework of tent poles over which the tent canvas could be spread. The makeshift tent stood four feet tall and hardly left room for sleeping-bags. Mawson made pannikins out of old ammunition tins; Mertz carved small wooden spoons.

Already the weakest dog had collapsed and been carried on the sledge. Now they killed it and skinned it. There was practically no fat, and what meat there was seemed tough and sinewy. A larger portion was fed to the dogs, who ate everything, crunching the bones and devouring even the skin. A smaller portion was put on one side for themselves; the rest they put into store. Now they had to prepare the meat. On this occasion they tried frying it, though this achieved little beyond scorching the outer surface. They found it had a strong musty flavour and was so stringy it was almost impossible to chew. Mawson noted: 'It was a happy relief when the liver appeared, even if little else could be said in its favour. It was easily chewed and demolished.'

It was now the southern midsummer and they found it better to camp by day and travel by night when temperatures were lower and the surface crisper. In a series of determined marches, they climbed steadily inland, hoping to find an easier route home south of the main body of glaciers. Over several days, despite the poor weather and the freshly fallen soft snow which hampered their steps, they averaged fifteen miles a day. But exhaustion and starvation were taking rapid toll of the dogs. Mawson developed snow-blindness and marched with one eye bandaged. Mertz walked by his side, since it was almost impossible for him to pull the sledge while on skis.

Christmas Day found them three quarters of the way across the Ninnis Glacier. At 160 miles from base camp, they had completed half their journey and were down to their last dog. One after another the animals had collapsed, pulling to the point of exhaustion. Stricken animals were carried on the sledge, but within a few hours Mawson and Mertz had had to kill them. More and more they needed to depend on the dog meat to conserve their ration packs as long as they could. They experimented with different ways of preparing the husky meat, such as chopping it finely, mixing it with a little pemmican and bringing it to the boil in a large pot of water. They found that if they boiled the meat very thoroughly they produced a tasty soup as well as a supply of edible meat in which the muscle and gristle were reduced to the consistency of jelly. The paws took the longest, but eventually, with lengthy stewing, even these became digestible. Yet it made repulsive eating.

Since it was Christmas they allowed themselves the luxury of one ounce of butter each to give the meal of dog stew a festive air. Mawson found a scrap of biscuit in the folds of his sleeping-bag, and they solemnly divided it between them.

They also further reduced the sledge load, jettisoning rifle and ammunition, camera and films, whether exposed or not. It was a silent acknowledgement of how slim their chances of survival had grown.

The next day they moved clear of the Ninnis Glacier and began climbing slowly across the vast terraces of the plateau. They had rigged a small sail for the sledge, using the skis as mast and boom and the tent canvas for a sail. Even so, progress remained painfully slow. Ginger, the last dog, was now incapable of pulling but trudged stoically alongside. After two days he gave in and collapsed, was carried on the sledge and finally killed. Even his brain, boiled in the skull, was scooped out and eaten in carefully apportioned spoonfuls.

During the early hours of 30 December they topped the last rise and stood on the exposed plateau uplands. Mawson described his feelings about the bleakness of the landscape with such phrases as 'the desolation of the outer worlds' and 'a solitude ominous yet weird'. The going here was easier, however, and Mawson and Mertz managed a determined march of fifteen miles before pitching tent. Yet now Mawson noticed for the first time that there was something disturbing in Mertz's manner. This naturally cheerful and talkative personality had fallen oddly silent. He was also wet and chilled, for his waterproof trousers had gone into the crevasse with the supplies and his clothing was penetrated and soaked through by the continual drift. No sooner was the tent up than Mertz crawled into his sleeping-bag and fell asleep. Mawson sat up for three hours, cooking more of the dog meat and pondering. 'Xavier off colour,' he noted briefly in his diary before crawling into his own sleeping-bag.

Within hours the weather had closed in, with thick drift and falling snow. They awoke to find everything in the tent caked with ice. The warmth of the prolonged bout of cooking had melted water frozen into the canvas and this had dripped over everything, soaked it, then refrozen. They peered out at the swirling maelstrom beyond the rattling canvas and retreated to the warmth of their sleeping-bags. Mertz was feeling a little better. In talking to Mawson, he confessed he thought the dog meat was not doing him much good and they decided to keep off it for a few days. Both were upset by it. In startling contrast, they found the normal rations tasted strangely sweet, but were so small in amount as to leave their stomachs painfully empty. Later in the day they attempted a march, but achieved no more than two and a half miles. A second attempt added five more miles, but they were forcing themselves through blinding drift. It was impossible to see where they were going and they were frightened of losing their direction. It was by now New Year's Eve.

On 1 January 1913, the weather was atrocious, heavily overcast with fierce driving winds and falling snow. Mertz was again off colour. He was miserable and silent, but complained only about the dampness of his sleeping-bag. When pressed by an anxious Mawson, he admitted he had pains in his stomach. Mawson was himself suffering from a continuous gnawing sensation in the abdomen and took it that Mertz felt the same discomfort, possibly more acutely. It seemed best to spend the day resting rather than blundering about in the bad light. As they lay crouched in their sleeping-bags Mertz suddenly expressed a craving for Glaxo; he had taken a dislike to biscuit. In an effort to help him, Mawson handed over their small store of Glaxo and accepted a considerable ration of dogs' meat in exchange. In the late evening they attempted to move on, but after a few miles Mertz was clearly distressed and they camped again.

The weather next day grew even worse, and they scarcely

stirred, contenting themselves with two ounces of chocolate each. If they were not travelling they could not afford to eat. The skin was now beginning to peel rapidly all over their bodies. At one point Mertz reached out and lifted a perfect skin cast from Mawson's ear, and Mawson was able to do the same for Mertz. This scaling of skin, known as desquamation, was particularly heavy on legs and genitalia. The new skin exposed seemed of poor quality which split readily and rubbed raw in many places. The hairs from every part of their bodies also became loose and fell out. Since they never removed their clothes, the peelings of skin and fallen hair worked down into their undertrousers and socks and regular clearances were needed.

On 3 January the clouds broke at last and the sun appeared. That evening they moved on, but the night air was so cold it gave Mertz frost-bite in his fingers and they were forced to make camp after only four and a half miles. Mertz now seemed in very poor condition. Large quantities of skin were peeling from his legs and he suddenly developed a 'dysentry', as Mawson termed it in his diary.

The next day dawned brighter and calmer than Mawson had dared to hope. Mertz's condition, however, seemed far worse. Reluctantly Mawson decided to let him spend the day resting. As Mertz lay silently in his sleeping-bag, Mawson worked fretfully at the gear, mending Mertz's clothing and cooking more of the dog meat. He broached one of the ration packs and served Mertz with milk. Towards midnight the snow returned and Mawson lay in his sleeping-bag, wrestling with a nagging desperation. The precious commodity time was slipping through their fingers.

The fifth of January was overcast with a moderate snowfall, though as morning progressed the weather calmed somewhat. Mawson was desperate to be on the move, but Mertz refused point-blank, saying it was suicide and that it was much better for him to spend another day in his sleeping-bag, drying it out and recouping his strength. They could do more once the sun was shining. Mawson tried to persuade him to attempt a mile or two, if only for the exercise. Outside in the 20 m.p.h. wind it was difficult to see far ahead. Eventually a compromise was reached. They would rest today, but on every day from tomorrow on would march. By tacit consent they had abandoned night travelling, and in the privacy of his diary Mawson expressed doubts about whether Mertz would in fact be able to move at all in the morning.

On 6 January the weather improved and the sun occasionally gleamed through the cloud. To Mawson's surprise, Mertz agreed to try a further march, but by now Mawson himself was feeling dizzy and weak, symptoms he attributed to the long stay in the sleeping-bags and lack of food. The surface they travelled over was good and they were moving downhill. At first Mertz walked slowly between long halts, but after two miles came to a dead stop. Following a brief argument he consented to ride on the sledge, and Mawson, aided by the makeshift sail, struggled to drag him another two and a half miles. Mertz was now so cold from inaction that there was no alternative but to make camp once more. Mertz, deeply depressed, after a brief meal settled down to sleep. But now his rest was uneasy. He seemed feverish and was again troubled by recurrent bouts of diarrhoea. He could not keep down the broth which Mawson attempted to feed him.

Reading between the lines of Mawson's diary for 6 January, it is clear that he felt a temptation to abandon Mertz – a temptation acknowledged and dismissed:

> things are in a most serious state for us both – if he cannot go 8 or 10 miles a day in a day or two we are doomed. I could pull myself

through with the provisions at hand – but I cannot leave him. His heart seems to have gone. It is very hard for me – to be within 100 miles of the hut and in such a position is awful.

And later:

A long wearisome night – if only I could get on – but I must stop with Xavier and he does not appear to be improving – both our chances are going now.

He awoke next morning, determined on a desperate march. He would carry Mertz, wrapped in his sleeping-bag, upon the sledge. But Mertz was in a terrible state. Too weak to move, he had fouled his trousers. He lay completely helpless as Mawson lifted him from his bag, struggled with the layers of clothing and worked at cleaning him up. At last he was clean and returned to the sleeping-bag to get warm. Mawson felt so cold and weak by now that he crept back into his own sleeping-bag for an hour before getting up to make another attempt. As he disturbed Mertz, however, he found him going into a kind of fit. Within a few minutes the convulsions stopped. Mertz came round and, exchanging a few words, seemed unaware of anything having happened.

As though to mock Mawson, the sun remained occasionally visible. The suppressed anguish in his diary is unmistakable:

Obviously we can't go on today – and it is a good day though bad light, the sun just gleaming through the clouds. This is terrible. I don't mind for myself but it is for Paquita and all the others connected with the expedition that I feel so deeply and sinfully – I pray God to help us.

He cooked beef tea and cocoa for Mertz and had to support him so he could drink it down. During the afternoon, Mertz went through several fits and became delirious. Again he was incontinent and again Mawson struggled with the task of cleaning him. The utmost gentleness of touch was called for, the skin over Mertz's legs and genitalia being raw and weeping. During the evening Mertz, confused and delirious, refused anything to eat or drink. At times he raved aloud, at others threw himself about so violently that he broke one of the tent-poles. Then he called, 'Oh, yea; oh, yea!' over and over for hours on end. Mawson struggled to hold him still in his sleeping-bag until, close on midnight, Mertz fell into a peaceful sleep. The exhausted Mawson crawled into his own sleeping-bag and drifted into a broken doze. Two hours later he awoke with the gradual realization that there had been no movement from his companion for some time. He stretched out an arm and found him cold and stiff. Xavier Mertz was dead.

For the rest of the night Mawson lay beside the corpse, his exhausted mind fumbling over and over the decisions forced upon him. By now he was struggling with a sense of isolation so immense it led to wonder and detachment. 'I seemed', he wrote, 'to stand alone on the shores of the wide world – and such a short step to enter the unknown future.' He was suddenly utterly overwhelmed by an urge to give in.

Outside there was nothing but intense cold, with ferocious, moaning winds worrying incessantly at everything beyond the tent's thin walls. He was at least a hundred miles from any other human being. He was too weak to pull the sledge alone. He was even uncertain whether, if he struck camp, he could ever find the strength to re-erect the tent single-handed. It seemed easier to sleep on in the relative warmth of his bag.

At 9 a.m., however, he forced himself up. As though declaring a momentary truce, the wind had fallen and he emerged into a calm world. Two simple lines from a poem by Robert Service had come into his head:

Buck up, do your damnedest and fight,
It's plugging away that will win you the day.

He would not give in; he would not lie supinely waiting for death. By now he hardly bothered to consider the chances of reaching base camp. Instead he rationalized his motives and reduced his aims. It would be something achieved to reach a prominent point as close to winter quarters as possible, where he might erect a cairn likely to catch the eye of a search party and there deposit both Mertz's and his own diaries. If there was no alternative to frozen oblivion, he would march to meet it.

His health had meanwhile deteriorated almost as rapidly as Mertz's. He felt perpetually on the verge of collapse. The skin of his legs and genitalia was raw; sores on his fingers refused to heal. Several toes were blackening and festering near the tips and the nails were working loose. Worst of all, the gnawing pains in his stomach increased and bent him double at times. The full weight of the sledge was beyond him. It took him most of one afternoon to cut it in two, chipping away at its wooden frame with a pocket knife. From the discarded half he retrieved rails to make a mast and spars for the truncated vehicle. Yet again he sifted the equipment, discarding as much as possible.

It was evening before he could bring himself to relinquish the physical presence of Mertz and drag from the tent the body still wrapped in its sleeping-bag. He piled snow blocks around it and bound together two discarded sledge runners to form a cross. At 10 p.m. he crept into his sleeping-bag and slept.

The following day the truce was over. Winds of 45 m.p.h.

swept the plateau. Philosophically, Mawson put aside all thoughts of travel. In his diary he began to note his own physical deterioration:

I have more to eat today in the hope that it will give me strength for the future. One annoying effect of the want of food is that wherever the skin breaks it refuses to heal – the nose and lips break open also – my scrotum, like Xavier's, is getting in a painfully raw condition due to reduced condition, dampness and friction in walking. It is well nigh impossible to treat.

That afternoon he stood beside Mertz's grave and read the funeral service aloud. In his diary he recorded the service and tried to give the bearings of the grave. The phrases virtually contained an apology for what he saw as his inevitable death and the failure of his mission:

as there is little chance of my reaching human aid alive, I greatly regret my inability to set out the coast line as surveyed for the 300 miles we travelled and the notes on glaciers and ice formations etc. – the most of which latter is of course committed to my head.

He was forced to confess he could not even be sure of the exact location of his camp.

The next day, 10 January, was impossible, with thick drift, high winds and practically no visibility. Once again Mawson occupied himself with simple tasks. He checked the food supplies and cooked all that remained of the dog meat. This chore completed, he made a calculated decision to abandon a large part of his stock of kerosene. It seemed impossible that he could survive to use it all. Towards evening the wind dropped at last, but he preferred to rest until morning, hoping his scrotum would heal.

On 11 January, a calm sunlit day, he struck camp. He packed his gear on to the half-sledge, stood a few silent moments beside Mertz's grave, then turned to challenge the

unvarying horizon. In no time at all he was in difficulties.
Within minutes his feet felt lumpy and sore. After a mile they
had grown so painful that he needed to sit on the sledge to
remove his shoes and socks. He found the soles of his feet
separated away as complete layers of thickened skin and his
socks saturated with fluid from the blisters. The newly
exposed skin was abraded and raw. He could think of nothing
but to smear his feet thickly with lanolin and bandage the
separated skin back on to each foot to act as an insole. He
donned six pairs of thick woollen socks beneath his fur boots
and struggled on for six and a half more miles.

Eventually exhausted, he made camp and cooked a meal.
His diary records his physical state:

> My whole body is apparently rotting from want of proper
> nourishment – frost-bitten fingertips, festerings, mucous membrane
> of nose gone, saliva glands of mouth refusing duty, skin coming off
> whole body.

In the morning his feet were too painful for walking and
he spent the time reviewing his food supplies and dividing
them into portions. He was annoyed to find himself contin-
ually nibbling fragments from different bags. The next day he
marched again, struggling down the ice-fields towards the
Mertz Glacier. At last he could see, in the far distance beyond
the glacier, the tip of Aurora Peak and the high uplands of
the plateau – the last great barrier that blocked the way to
Commonwealth Bay and the huts of base camp.

Once again he began to pick up a path between the
treacherous crevasses of the Mertz Glacier. On the third day
on the glacier a close to final disaster struck when a snow-
bridge collapsed. He found himself hanging fourteen feet
down in the dark cold of a crevasse whose massive ice walls,
barely six feet apart, plunged into blackness. The rope on

which he hung was slipping as the sledge, high above, crept in little jerks towards the edge of the crevasse. 'So this is the end,' he thought and waited. Nothing happened. With instinctive regret his mind went to the carefully hoarded food which remained uneaten on the sledge, until gradually he grew aware that he was spinning slowly round on the end of the rope. The rope had sawn into the overlaying crust of snow; the sledge had stopped moving.

But now the cold and pain hit him. Since it was a warm day, he had removed his gloves before the mishap. The ends of his fingers were damaged and raw; several pounds of dislodged snow had forced its way inside his clothing. A razor-sharp chill cut into every part of his body.

The rope had a series of knots and it took a desperate effort to bring one knot within his grasp. Slowly he fought his way upwards, dragging himself from knot to knot until his head and shoulders emerged above the crust and he lay for a moment sobbing for breath in the relative warmth of the sun. But even as he struggled to draw himself completely out, the snow lid gave way and he fell again with a sickening shock as the rope snatched and held firm, suspending him even lower in the dark and cold. For some minutes he struggled ineffectually, trying to haul himself up, but then he hung silently battling with a sudden temptation simply to slip from the harness and let himself drop.

In the end he stirred. He had the strength left for no more than one last attempt. Clawing his way upwards in what seemed an eternity of agonizing muscle spasms and tearing, weeping skin, he neared the top, leant his body backwards and drove his feet and legs out first along the track of the rope. Then, slithering stomach-down on the snow crust, he inched slowly away from the brim. The moment he knew he was lying on firm ground a reaction set in and for an hour he could do no more. Eventually, in slow stages, he erected his tent, gnawed at a little food, crawled into his bag and slept. It was early afternoon.

He awoke to yet another day of temptation: this time to lie in his tent, eat through his entire food supply and enjoy life for a few days rather than fight on in wretched hunger, only to plunge to sudden death- in a crevasse and leave food uneaten. His inner turmoil was increased by knowing that the outside world could only now be growing aware that he might be in trouble. He was just two days overdue at base camp.

Instead of broaching his stores, however, he lay in his sleeping-bag and constructed a makeshift rope-ladder from an alpine rope. One end was to be anchored to the sledge, the other carried loosely over his shoulder and attached to his harness. If he fell into a crevasse again and the sledge held firm, he should then be able to climb out with ease. The following day he reduced his rations still further, marched again, and discovered that the ladder worked when it retrieved him from another plunge.

His feet were now in a pitiful state. Much time needed to be spent each day dressing and redressing them. On 19 January, a day on which he achieved a distance of only three and a half miles but cleared the western rim of the Mertz Glacier, he noted in his diary: 'I took off all clothes to get to boil on leg and stuck it.' With his physical problems and the overriding sense of weakness, he was managing to maintain average marches of only about four miles a day and had lost several days pinned down by blizzards and blinding weather.

Now his path lay uphill, past Aurora Peak on to the last great plateau between him and Commonwealth Bay. He calculated he must be within sixty-five miles of the hut. As he climbed he jettisoned yet more equipment, throwing away his alpine rope, the crevasse stick and worn-out crampons. His movements were hampered by soft wet snow which dragged at his legs and feet and clung to the sledge runners. On the plateau itself, violent squalls of freezing wind repeatedly capsized the sledge and filled his goggles with snow. On 24 January he referred to the state of his hands: 'Both my hands have shed the skin in large sheets; it is a great nuisance and very tender.'

The following day he was pinned down yet again, this time by storm winds strong enough to blow away a number of packages left in the open. Deep falls of fresh snow crushed in the walls of the tent until it was reduced to about the dimensions of a coffin. The chill simile occurred to him as he lay in his sleeping-bag, and he shuddered at it. On 26 January, he summoned up courage, struck camp in 60 m.p.h. winds, marched nearly eight miles and then fought for two hours to re-erect the tent. For days his hair had been dropping so that the snowy floor of the tent was strewn with it. In his diary on 27 January 1913 he commented:

For the last 2 days my hair has been falling out in handfuls and rivals the reindeer hair from the moulting bag for nuisance – In all food preparations. My beard on one side has come out in patches.

Two days later he spent an hour and a half digging sledge and tent free from the snow which buried them. As he marched, the weather began to clear and he realized he was travelling gently downhill. He had crossed the crest of the 3,000-foot-high plateau and was beginning the long descent to the coast. As the sky brightened, he made out, forty miles away, a dark patch between the flat horizon and the great piles of cumulus cloud. It was the indented coastline of Commonwealth Bay. He was within distant sight of base camp.

The evening was given over to feverish calculations. He must be within thirty-five perhaps even thirty miles of Aladdin's Cave and its treasure of provisions. At his present rate of progress he could not hope to reach it in less than eight or nine days. There were just two pounds of food left. Could he accomplish such a journey on daily rations as meagre as three or four ounces?

The following day the weather closed in and Commonwealth Bay vanished as though it had never existed. For five miles he trudged steadily downhill through brisk winds and an obscuring drift. At 2 p.m. he made out something dark 300 yards to the north of his path and turned towards it. It was a piece of black cloth stretched across a cairn of rough-hewn snow-blocks. On the top of the cairn lay a bag of provisions and a small tin box, left by a relief party out searching for him.

The astonishing fact was that Mawson had taken forty-six days to drive himself on foot nearly 300 miles through the worst wilderness known to man, navigating by means of a damaged theodolite balanced on the corner of the cooker box, a compass rendered unreliable by the proximity of the South Magnetic Pole and a watch which had stopped at least two or three times. Though he kept a careful tally of his estimates for his daily marches, he had been reckoning progress by a sledge cyclometer that repeatedly jammed and broke. Yet here he was returning to base within 300 yards of his predicted line of travel.

In the tin box, Mawson found a brief note from the relief expedition. They had built the cairn, cached the bag of provisions and were now returning to base. The expedition ship *Aurora* had already arrived to evacuate the party and was waiting to sail. There was news: Amundsen had reached the South Pole; Scott was still somewhere in the Antarctic.

The note went on to give an exact bearing relative to Aladdin's Cave, in fact twenty-three miles distant. It was signed and dated, and with a sense of shock Mawson realized the relief expedition had left the cairn barely six hours before. He had spent the night camped within five miles of help.

While the diary gives little indication of any reaction, Mawson's emotional turmoil may be gauged by the difficulty he now experienced deciphering the bearings, given as S.60.E., and choosing the correct line of march. For half a mile he trudged on the compass bearings before realizing he was travelling directly away from his goal. He retraced his steps, calculating his direction in his confusion as N.30.W. Only after a mile and a half of pondering on the problem did he turn to his true bearing of N.60.W., and even then his instincts rebelled against the decision, trying to convince him that this path lay too far west. As he struggled down the vast ice-fields he worried over whether or not the relief expedition could have observed or recorded the bearings correctly, while in his pursuit of the relief party the weather and terrain seemed intent on thwarting him. The soft snow had been replaced by iron-hard ice, frozen into irregular ridges. Lacking crampons, he slipped and fell again and again. Each blast of wind seemed able to sweep his legs from under him.

He used his new rations cautiously, disciplining himself so that no sudden increase in diet should upset his stomach. An improvement in stamina was, however, immediately apparent. Despite all obstacles he was making excellent progress, covering thirteen and a half miles in the day.

On 30 January he improvised crampons, dismantling the sledge meter for its screws and tacks, which he drove into pieces of wood cut from the theodolite box. With the make-shift crampons lashed to his feet he laboured on, but not until two days later, at seven in the evening of 2 February, did he find the beacon marking the entrance to Aladdin's Cave and stumble into its shelter. In the very centre of the floor lay a small heap of fruit: three oranges and a pineapple. For the first time during his ordeal he wept, kneeling and overcome by the sight of something unwhite.

There were only five further miles to base camp, but the weather, as if in one last furious effort to claim him, deteriorated into an unrelenting blizzard worse than anything hitherto encountered. For an entire week he rested secure in Aladdin's Cave as the gales tore at the ice-fields above his head. He improvised fresh crampons, his makeshift pair having disintegrated. He even began to puzzle over his condition, recognizing that something curious had been happening to his body.

In his diary for 3 February 1913 he noted:

I turned in at midnight very tired – it almost appears as if scurvy or something of the kind were upon me – joints very sore. Blood keeps coming from my right nostril in thin watery description – also from outburst on the fingers.

In his perplexed frame of mind, he was even suspicious of the food supplies left for him. 'Am quite sure some of the food here is overstale,' he wrote. 'I may be getting hurt from it.' But the question that occupied his thoughts most was whether the expedition would have waited. The *Aurora* had been due to sail a fortnight before, when the relief expedition began its search.

At last, on 8 February, the wind lessened enough for him to leave Aladdin's Cave. Early in the afternoon he began the last stage of his journey, but as he neared base camp could see no sign of the ship. Then he caught sight of her far out to sea, a distant shape steaming slowly for the northern horizon. The hut itself looked silent and deserted as he approached, but suddenly there came a flicker of movement, and all at once he picked out three men working close to the boat harbour. A shore party had been left to wait.

The story of Douglas Mawson's return from the obliviating wastes of Antarctica is one of the major epics of survival in the annals of exploration. He preserved his life and brought back not only himself but the scientific knowledge gained and a battered diary with its scribbled entries. This diary contained, in effect, a strange specimen: an account of a disease which would continue to baffle medical scientists for more than half a century.

When Mawson reached base hut on 8 February 1913, he was a shadow of the man who set out. His weight was down from 15 to 8 stone. His appearance was so changed that the colleagues who ran to meet him found it difficult in the first fleeting moment to recognize which member of the Far-Eastern Sledge Party survived.

The *Aurora*, on receiving the news by radio, attempted to turn back, but could make no headway in the face of the southerly gales. Thus Mawson and the relief party found themselves condemned to yet another Antarctic winter. The prolonged, enforced period of rest was probably a godsend for Mawson, however. In his diary he wrote:

I was overcome with a soft and smooth feeling of thanksgiving. At first stumbling, then as the tension relaxed a day or two after I began to feel the whole weight of the privations endured . . .

On 11 February he noted: 'My legs have now swollen very much . . .' The next day he remarked: 'I have shaken to pieces somewhat.' At first he did little except potter, eat and doze. From his companions he received a concern he found moving. They, in turn, noticed how he followed them around, not so much to talk as just to be with them. It was several weeks before normal sleep returned, and for almost two months his days and nights were disturbed by frequent attacks of diarrhoea.

He used the radio, in short snatches through intense static interference, to send messages announcing his survival, messages to the families of Ninnis and Mertz, and a message asking for royal assent to his proposal to call the land he had travelled through King George V Land. But his sense of failure endured. To Paquita he sent a heartbreaking telegram, announcing his escape but humbly offering to release her from her engagement.

By now he was falling prey to an unfamiliar nervous tension and aware of ever-increasing emotional disturbance. On 27 March he wrote:

I find my nerves in a serious state, and from the feeling I have in the back of my head I suspicion that I may go off my rocker very soon. My nerves have evidently had a very great shock. Too much writing today has brought this on. I shall take more exercise and less study hoping for a beneficial turn.

His fears for his sanity were real, but as his physical condition improved, so his agitation settled and the slow months of the Antarctic winter saw a gradual return to natural equanimity and resilience. He still suffered, however, from occasional delayed physical effects of his ordeal. On 27 May he was still writing: 'I have a boil on the left temple forming. Am quite down in general health.' Whatever the disease was that afflicted him, it took several months to relinquish its grip and leave him in peace.

The questions raised were simply ones of diagnosis. What had been the strange disorder which overtook the Far-Eastern Sledge Party, killed Xavier Mertz and virtually reduced

Douglas Mawson to the status of an emotional and physical invalid? The pages of Mawson's diary furnish a superb description, and few physicians at a patient's bedside could hope to have so lucid and comprehensive a case-history on which to reach a conclusion. Unfortunately, no diagnosis was forthcoming.

Mawson expressed the impression that Mertz's death was caused by 'exposure, finally bringing on a fever, result of weather, exposure and want of food'. Undoubtedly hypothermia and semi-starvation were contributory factors, but death from either cause is preceded by inertia and coma, not by violent delirium and convulsions; certainly not by desquamation or hair loss. Scurvy was one cause which Mawson himself considered, but that well-documented condition could be dismissed out of hand in the light of the clinical picture.

The disease which Mawson described had an insidious onset, beginning with lethargy, general weakness and depression. Its most remarkable symptoms, the generalized desquamation of the skin and loss of hair, then followed. There was a disturbance of the appetite, abdominal pains, diarrhoea, muscle and joint pain, nose-bleeds and swollen legs; and in the acute fulminating case of the unfortunate Dr Mertz, confusion, convulsions, delirium and death.

The irony of it was that clues already existed, but lay literally a world away. They were not in any scientific archives or medical data sheets, but in travellers' tales from the Arctic Circle and Eskimo folklore. Over 300 years before, Gerrit de Veer had published *The True and Perfect Description of Three Voyages so Strange and Wonderful the Like Hath Never Been Heard Before: The Navigation into the Northe Seas, etc.* (London, 1609). It contained an account of the Dutch Expedition of 1596, led by William Barents, which was forced to winter at Novaya

Zemlya. On 31 May 1597, some of the party, driven by hunger, took the liver of a polar bear they had killed,

> and drest and eate it; the taste liked us well, but it made us all sicke, especially three that were exceeding sicke, and we verily thought that we should have lost them for all their skins came off from foote to heade; but yet they recovered again, for which we gave God heartie thanks, for if as then we had lost these three men, it was a hundred to one that we should have had too few men to draw and lift at our neade.

Gerrit de Veer concluded that the polar-bear liver had poisoned them, and this was no isolated observation. Practically every Arctic explorer of the nineteenth century brought back tales of similar curious disorders following the eating of polar-bear liver.

The most graphic account came from the Denmark Expedition of 1907. On 10 March, a polar bear was shot from the deck of the ship. The following day a ragout was prepared from the bear's liver. It was eaten by nineteen men, including the expedition's medical officer, Dr Lindhard, who chronicled what followed. All nineteen fell ill. Within a few hours they were struggling against an irresistible desire to sleep. Soon they were suffering severe headaches, a deep-seated hammering or boring pain made worse by movement or coughing or sneezing. After reaching a climax, the headaches slowly subsided and disappeared within a day or two. Three men suffered from convulsions: episodes of rigid muscle spasm followed by violent jerking of the limbs. Most suffered loss of appetite, nausea or persistent bouts of vomiting. Several complained of shivering as if in a fever, though their temperatures were subnormal. In ten patients there was widespread peeling of the skin, and in one unfortunate individual this continued for more than a month.

In Eskimo tradition the liver of the polar bear was always taboo. Misfortune in the probable shape of illness, it was believed, would strike at anyone who ate it. The livers of the bearded seal, Arctic shark and Arctic fox were regarded with almost equal wariness. Even so, no scientific reasons for toxic qualities in polar-bear liver were sought before 1939, when a young Norwegian medical investigator, Dr Kaara Rodahl, joined a party of scientists who spent the winter of 1939–40 making biological observations at a laboratory established at Rerct, a trappers' station in north-east Greenland. During the winter he managed to collect among other specimens the complete livers of two polar bears. He packed his specimens in a barrel of brine to preserve them until he could get them back to Norway for analysis, but in the spring of 1940 Germany invaded his country. Thus Rodahl, with his barrel of specimens, arrived in England at Cambridge University as a refugee scientist.

Preliminary studies of the livers yielded perplexing results. No unexpected substances or poisons could be discovered. Their one unusual characteristic seemed to be that they carried a remarkably rich store of vitamin A. It was present in concentrations about a hundred times greater than usual in the livers of such domestic animals as the ox or the lamb. The liver of a third polar bear, collected for Rodahl by the Norwegian Arctic Patrol during the winter of 1940–41, simply confirmed these findings. The livers of two bearded seals similarly showed nothing out of the ordinary beyond intense concentrations of vitamin A.

The intriguing possibility now arose that poisoning by polar-bear liver could, in fact, be vitamin A overdosage. Armed with this hypothesis, Rodahl set out to test it in the laboratory. It proved an unexpectedly difficult undertaking. Most of the rats used in the experiment refused the liver, and only five rats ate any. Three of these showed no ill effects; two became ill and one of them died.

Rodahl now fractionalized the liver and tried to feed varying extracts of tissue to his rats. Once again the results were conflicting. When, in 1943, he eventually wrote up his experiments with his co-worker, T. Moore, for an article in the journal *Nature*, they were able to do no more than postulate that polar-bear-liver poisoning might be caused by ingesting excessive vitamin A.

After the war, in 1947, Kaara Rodahl was offered a place on the Danish Airborne Expedition to Peary Land in north-east Greenland. He returned this time with specimens of liver not only from polar bears and seals but from a wide variety of Arctic mammals, birds and fish. The interesting fact emerged that high concentrations of vitamin A occurred not merely in the polar bear and bearded seal, but in every Arctic animal in which the liver was reputedly poisonous. He also made a converse discovery. Animals, like the walrus and Arctic hare, which the Eskimos considered safe to eat had low concentrations in their livers.

By now he had succeeded in developing his techniques in his animal trials and was able to make a series of conclusive observations. First, a daily intake of polar-bear liver or of extracted liver oil invariably caused illness in rats, sometimes fatal. Second, polar-bear liver or the oil did no harm once it was free of its vitamin A content. The degree of illness produced was directly in proportion to the dose given, and an equivalent dose of vitamin A from other sources produced identical symptoms. It was beyond dispute that the toxic effects known to the Eskimos and stumbled over by generations of Arctic travellers were caused by overdosage of vitamin A.

In fact, the polar bear was the last link in a food chain which led to an accumulation and concentration of vitamin A with every step. At the outset the vitamin A was formed in plankton in the sea. The plankton was consumed by fishes, which concentrated and stored the vitamin in their livers; hence the richness of cod-liver oil and halibut-liver oil. The fishes were then eaten by seals; the seals were eaten by polar bears. As small a quantity as three or four ounces of polar-bear liver could contain enough vitamin A to bring on acute illness.

By the time Rodahl published his work, however, vitamin A poisoning was a well-recognized disorder christened hypervitaminosis A. Concentrations of vitamin A had become commercially available and a number of vitamin enthusiasts fell foul of their enthusiasm by overdosing themselves. Some doctors also prescribed it for certain conditions, unaware that a vitamin could cause poisoning. The first cases of hypervitaminosis A were recognized in children as early as 1944; the first adult case was described in 1951. By the 1960s and early 1970s a reasonably comprehensive clinical picture had emerged. Two different states of intoxication were recognizable: first, an acute poisoning from a single, very large dose; and second, a chronic form where excessive doses had been taken at regular intervals over a long period.

In the acute variety, the symptoms were fairly consistent. Abdominal pain, nausea, vomiting, severe headache, sluggishness, irritability and a strong desire to sleep came on inside a few hours. Within a day or two there would be generalized peeling of the skin and then, usually, a gradual recovery over the course of two or three days.

Chronic intoxication was rather more insidious. It was remarkably difficult to diagnose in adults, and victims often suffered many medical fumblings before the cause was brought to light. The clinical picture was highly variable.

Drying of the skin with fissuring, often about the mouth, and widespread peeling seemed general. There might be a rash or pigmentation, and occasionally some itching. Hair loss could be from the scalp only, or might include all body hair. Weakness and fatigue, with tenderness or pain in the bones or joints, were common symptoms, as were nausea and loss of appetite and weight. Severe headache could be a feature in about half the patients, and it took a while for it to be realized how, by raising intracranial pressure, vitamin A intoxication could exactly mimic the clinical picture for a cerebral tumour, one or two patients actually suffering unnecessary brain surgery as neurosurgeons probed for a non-existent growth. Mental health could also deteriorate in ways ranging from mild depression to an acute breakdown which needed treatment in a psychiatric unit.

Only in 1969 did it occur to anyone to ask whether Xavier Mertz and Douglas Mawson could have been victims of hypervitaminosis A. In that year Professor Sir John Cleland of the University of Adelaide and Dr R. V. Southcott, a zoologist, put forward the suggestion that they had contracted it by eating the livers of their husky dogs. The Arctic husky is among the animals whose livers are incriminated by Eskimo folklore, and Cleland and Southcott suggested that all the symptoms suffered by Mertz and Mawson during the epic march across King George V Land had fitted the typical clinical picture of acute vitamin A intoxication in the first case, and sub-acute or chronic intoxication in the second.

Mertz's convulsions, delirium and eventual coma all suggested a raised intracranial pressure, the pseudo-'cerebral tumour' syndrome. Severe vitamin A intoxication can produce a tendency to haemorrhage, and in experimental animals, at least, intractable diarrhoea has occasionally resulted from small haemorrhages into the walls of the intestine.

Possibly this could have accounted for his diarrhoea and eventual incontinence.

On the other hand, the story of Douglas Mawson presented a virtually complete compendium of the symptoms of sub-acute or chronic hypervitaminosis A. Cleland and Southcott could think of no other explanation to account so adequately for all the facets of his illness. They went on to compare the two explorers' situation with that which had faced others, such as Nansen and Amundsen. Amundsen's expedition to the South Pole in 1912 had deliberately used its dog teams both for transport and to provide food. Nansen and Amundsen were alike aware of Eskimo folklore and of the dangers of eating the livers of Arctic animals. In his own account of the discovery of the South Pole, Amundsen wrote, 'if we . . . wanted a piece of fresh meat we could cut off from the dog carcass a delicate little fillet, it tasted to us as good as the best beef'. It seems that only lean dog meat was eaten by these explorers, the livers and entrails being fed to the other dogs.

The one difficulty with this hypothesis lay in the fact that nobody had measured the vitamin A content in the liver of huskies transported to Antarctica. In 1971, to test Cleland's and Southcott's proposal, specimens of liver were collected from huskies at the Antarctic bases of the Australian National Antarctic Research Expedition (ANARE). In every specimen the vitamin A concentration was remarkably high. On average, about 100 grams (3 ounces) of husky liver were found to contain a toxic dose of vitamin A.

A single question remained to be answered. Why did Mertz suffer from such an acute fulminating intoxication while Mawson showed the sub-acute or chronic form? In 1978, Professor Shearman, Professor of Medicine at Adelaide University, suggested that Mawson may have allowed Mertz, a near vegetarian, to take the lion's share of the liver, which was more easily eaten and digested than the meat. This informed guess looks as close to an explanation as we are likely to arrive.

One telegram in particular had been repeatedly transmitted through the auroral static until safely received at Commonwealth Bay and handed to Mawson. It was the reply from Paquita:

DEEPLY THANKFUL YOU ARE SAFE STOP WARMEST WELCOME AWAITING YOUR HAIRLESS RETURN STOP REGARDING CONTRACT SAME AS EVER ONLY MORE SO STOP THOUGHTS ALWAYS WITH YOU STOP . . .

A Mawson Relief Fund had been set up in England and Australia, which enabled the *Aurora* to make a rescue voyage and take Mawson and his shore party off Commonwealth Bay in December 1913. Even so Mawson remained determined that they should chart from the sea one last great arc of coastline before sailing north for Australia. He was first and foremost a dedicated scientist, determined to complete the job he set out to achieve. He was an impressive figure, but flamboyant heroism was not his style.

When he returned to Australia, apart from marrying his Paquita he set about lecturing, making personal appearances and writing an account so as to raise the money to clear the deficit which remained in the expedition's funds. Official honours were never lacking: a knighthood in 1914; the Founders' Medal of the Royal Geographical Society in 1915; the OBE in 1920. In 1923 he was elected a Fellow of the Royal Society, and his career continued as a geologist of great distinction. Yet, in the public mind, neither he nor the astonishing story of his survival against desperate hazards received the fame they deserved. His epic achievement remained overshadowed by the drama of the tragic outcome of the Scott expedition, the frozen bodies of Scott's party having been discovered on 12 November 1912, only two days after Mawson set out. And then, within a few months of his return to Australia, the infinitely vaster tragic drama of the First World War broke in Europe.

Sir Douglas Mawson died in Adelaide in 1958 at the age of seventy-six, and was given a state funeral. He was acknowledged as having been among the very front rank of Antarctic explorers. The school of geology in Adelaide had been named after him, and in 1961 the Mawson Institute of Antarctic Research was set up to carry on his work. He was largely instrumental in claiming the vast tracts of the Australian Antarctic Territory for his country, and the first permanent scientific station to be set up there by Australia was called Mawson. The most moving tribute to his memory must, however, be a treasured exhibit which stands in the South Australia Museum on permanent loan from the Royal Geographical Society of London: the battered half of the last sledge.

The story of vitamin A continues to unravel and the understanding of hypervitaminosis A has assumed new significance. Patients with chronic kidney failure often carry high levels of vitamin A in their blood, and the possible risk of vitamin intoxication in patients on artificial kidney machines has been recognized and avoided. Vitamin A itself holds out a promise of great rewards, for it has long been realized that it can in high doses prevent or even cure cancer formation in certain tissues. Once a way is discovered of preventing intoxication from high doses, vitamin A could in the future become an important weapon in our anti-cancer armoury. Experiments suggest that it should eventually be possible to modify the side-effects.

Douglas Mawson, of course, never knew what the cause had been of the illness which struck at the Far-Eastern Sledge Party. He would no doubt have appreciated, if with a certain wry irony, how knowledge of the malady unexpectedly supported his own scientific philosophy. From the beginning he maintained that information wrested from the remote and frozen wastes of Antarctica would in the long run have relevance for the lives of everyone on this planet.

Chapter 13

The Balkan Enigma

There exist, in the world of medicine, infinitely more disconcerting puzzles than there are explanations to fit them. It is therefore only right that this fact should be acknowledged, and it would be hard to illustrate it more graphically than with the problem of the Balkan nephropathy. As with all true mysteries, the explanation must look simple, even inevitable, once it is understood, yet it has, for over thirty years, continued to defy detection.

The Bulgarian authorities were the first to become aware of something drastically wrong when, in 1950, officials of the Bulgarian Ministry of Public Health and Social Welfare received a disturbing report. A very curious thing seemed to be happening in the small villages which lay in the northern foothills of the Balkan Mountains, in the country's extreme north-west corner. The population there appeared to be suffering from a bizarre, even unique, outbreak of kidney disease. To put it statistically there were, quite simply, too many people dying from renal failure.

The region indicated was a hilly area of pasture and farmland, with small villages and hamlets dotted here and there and fast-flowing rivers hurrying northwards down to the vast flood-plain of the Danube. The main town of the district was Vratza, which, with its 45,000 inhabitants, served as the regional administrative centre as well as a garrison town. It was also an important rail junction and possessed several thriving industries, including a giant chemical complex powered by natural gas. Oddly enough, the people of the town seemed totally unaffected by the trouble which had attracted a team of medical investigators. Whatever was happening appeared to be a problem strictly of the countryside, a rural rather than an urban blight.

A series of large-scale surveys over the following weeks defined the area affected: a limited tract in the foothills, about seventy kilometres long by thirty or so kilometres wide. It contained two other towns besides Vratza, and seventy-seven villages. Nothing abnormal came to light in any of the towns, but fifty-two villages revealed undeniable evidence of an increased incidence of kidney disease. In fourteen villages it had virtually reached epidemic proportions.

The figures which the doctors produced were startling. In an average European or North American community, 1 per cent of deaths occurring may perhaps be attributed to kidney disease; for Bulgaria in general the figure was, in fact, 1·2 per cent. A survey of the villages about Vratza, however, revealed that 34 per cent of all deaths were caused by kidney disease. In some villages, as many as 12 per cent of the inhabitants had an advanced kidney condition and early symptoms were suspected in another 25 per cent. In other words, in certain villages over a third of the villagers were either proven or suspected cases. And, as if this were not enough, doctors were hesitantly suggesting that the unparalleled outbreak was caused, not by any sudden increase in one of the commonly occurring conditions, but by an entirely new disorder, a previously unrecognized form of kidney complaint.

The chronic diseases which afflict the kidney tend, as a group, to have anonymous faces and unobtrusive disposi-

tions. It is rare for them to advertise by any dram
outward indication the desperate circumstances developing
behind the scenes. The bystander may notice almost nothing;
even the patient may remain unaware of any ailment until its
smouldering on over many years has produced dangerous
and irretrievable kidney damage. With the clinical presenta-
tions being so inconspicuous, it can be difficult to distinguish
between one kidney disease and another, and it may take an
experienced physician with the support of a battery of
investigations to assess the degree of renal damage in a
patient and disentangle a correct diagnosis out of the long
list of disorders known to attack the kidney. The task
of recognizing and defining any previously undescribed
kidney disease therefore demands a cautious, unhasty approach.

Yet, despite their natural reservations and hesitations, the
medical research teams were building up a distinctive but
unfamiliar clinical picture of an insidious disease that crept
up on the sufferer as a lethargy, a sense of tiredness and
weakness in the lumbar region. Some patients complained of
abdominal discomfort, constipation, an aching in limbs and
joints, headaches, or the passage of large amounts of urine;
the more general experience, however, was of a vague, slow
loss of appetite and weight which faded into a gradual but
profound anaemia that could only be relieved by regular
blood transfusions. Observers from Western medical centres
watched startled as patients, outwardly well in every other
respect, were temporarily rejuvenated by transfusions and
left the clinic to return to their rural labours. One of the more
singular features of the disease was a pale coppery-yellow
sheen which appeared on the facial skin, most noticeably in
the spring and autumn. The palms of the hands and the soles
of the feet also tended to develop an ochre discolouration.

But, despite these outward signs, the disease was usually overlooked till far advanced.

Paradoxically, the disorder was in some ways more remarkable for the symptoms and complications it did not possess but which are common features of other renal diseases. The urine was not, for example, heavily laden with albumin since there was only a relatively slight leakage of protein from the kidney. There was no sign of fluid retention in the body's tissues or of raised blood pressure, and not the slightest evidence of damage to blood vessels, eyes or bones.

The most striking feature of the disease was perhaps the sharply defined group which it seemed to attack. Its victims were middle-aged between thirty and sixty, and included men and women, though women were maybe more affected. A child or younger person with the illness was a rarity. All the patients were directly involved with the land as agricultural workers, farmers, their wives and families. Those occasional individuals who lived in the villages but followed some other occupation, such as teaching, seemed to be immune.

For experienced observers the most unexpected finding was that it had the look of a familial disease. The disorder concentrated itself in households and there were homes where two, three or even more members of the household had contracted it. There were families in which husband and wife and eventually all their grown-up children displayed its unmistakable signs. There were even families where it could be recognized in three generations.

By now the researchers had unearthed over 3,000 cases, each one of which proved to be tragically progressive. It could be anticipated that each patient would, within two to three years of a diagnosis, be sunk in a state of severe renal failure leading to inevitable uraemia and death. Kidneys examined at autopsy were found to be shrivelled to a third or even a quarter of their natural size. But what could the cause be, and what was so special about this one small region of the Balkan foothills that it should generate such a hazard for its inhabitants?

Geologically speaking, the region lay in a syncline built mainly of Lower Cretaceous sandstones, limestone, clayey marls and Upper Cretaceous limestones. The most typical characteristic of the rock and soil content was a high concentration of phosphorus combined with traces of lead, copper, zinc, barium and several other elements. The region was hardly geologically unique, however, and the same syncline supported three towns and at least two dozen villages in which no trace of the disease existed. The irregular distribution of the disease within the area was itself intriguing, and it was noticeable how it occurred mainly in villages which lay in the floors of the valleys and along the banks of the rivers. Similar villages which lay nearby but happened to perch on a hilltop or high up a hillside looking down into the valleys escaped untouched. From the viewpoint of altitude, it was possible to say that the disease only occurred in villages which lay between 150 and 300 metres above sea-level. Even then, individual villages contained curious anomalies. Practically every house down one side of a particular street might be the home of patients suffering from the disease, while their neighbours opposite remained completely healthy. The local inhabitants themselves spoke of 'black houses' and the unfortunate histories of certain villages. The investigators were utterly lost for an explanation.

As first reports of the disease reached publication, events took an unexpected turn. There was news from Romania.

Across the border, just over eighty kilometres to the north-west of Vratza, on the far side of the flood-plain of the Danube where the Carpathians sweep down in undulating hills to reach the river at Turnu Severin, another pocket of the disease emerged. Again, it appeared to be restricted to a sharply circumscribed region and to involve only rural communities. Again, the disease occurred exclusively among the middle-aged and predominantly among those who worked on the land. Again, altitude seemed to bestow immunity.

In this region of the Balkan peninsula, close to the 'Bend of the Danube' where the river breaks through the mountains to reach its flood-plain, the territories of both Romania and Bulgaria are bordered to the west by Yugoslavia. And now, to confound matters even further, several small isolated out-breaks of the disease were discovered, all scattered along tributaries of the Danube, in various Yugoslav provinces. In Serbia, on the opposite side of the Balkan Mountains from Vratza, there was a pocket in the foothills along the valley of the Morava, and another in the valley of the Kolubara. In Bosnia, there was a small outbreak in the valley of the Drina, and yet another along the banks of the Sava, from Bjelina all the way up to Slavonski Brod in Croatia. In each region the disease was confined to quite a limited area and once more displayed all its puzzling features. Over 20,000 cases were on record by this stage.

The discovery of these different areas of infection compli-cated the problem. The jigsaw now had several pieces, none of which seemed to interlock. Somewhere there must be a com-mon feature which united these separate areas yet set them apart from the rest of the world. All had been discovered almost simultaneously. They were clustered, with barely 100 to 150 kilometres separating one pocket of the disease from another, in a small group at the very centre of the Balkan peninsula.

Geographically, it was clear that they each occurred in the floor of a mountain valley at the point of transition between valley and plain. Each shared the same Mediterranean climate, high humidity and hot, close summers contrasting with the long, bitterly cold winters of the mountains. All were in regions rich in vegetation, where trees such as the Turkish hazel, the Spanish sweet chestnut and the wild walnut could flourish. Wildlife was varied and plentiful with foxes, wildcats, squirrels, several species of rodent, vipers and even bears; in Bulgaria, another twenty years would pass before the wolf was declared an endangered species.

The villages were picturesque and primitive. At least 70 per cent of houses had one or more rooms with dirt floors. There were unhygienic privies and dunghills, and hosts of flies and mosquitoes. Water came from wells. For the villager, life was simple and impoverished, sustained mainly by the daily struggle of subsistence farming. Working conditions were poor, and in bad weather even the simplest agricultural tasks required considerable effort. Winter brought the extra ordeals of almost constant wet and biting cold. Tuberculosis was common and outbreaks of typhoid and dysentery were not infrequent. Malaria was just being brought under control. Yet these unpleasant aspects of life were general throughout the region and shared alike by affected and unaffected villages. There was nothing in them to explain the distribution of the disease.

The very harshness of life in the villages made it hard to estimate how long the disease had existed. Balkan nephropathy attacked individuals between the ages of thirty and sixty, but as late as 1940 the average expectation of life for a farmer in the region was still only forty years. Very few survived to be sixty-five. The villagers themselves could recall whole families being afflicted by a fatal disease as long as twenty or thirty years earlier, and church records from before the Second World War confirmed that it was not infrequent for several members of a family to die young. Unfortunately, such records gave no details of the causes of death, but at least one doctor who had worked in the Vratza region in his youth in 1941–2 remembered many people dying from kidney failure.

Almost all the Yugoslav church records had been destroyed during the Second World War, but the priests were certain that there had been many people dying from kidney disease even before the First World War. Neither the priests nor the local doctors, however, could define the exact nature of this disease. The story was confirmed by Volhard, the German physiologist, who noted that German doctors had, while working in Serbia in 1915 during the German occupation, reported large numbers of deaths from uraemia. It looked as though Balkan nephropathy had been smouldering on in the region for at least forty years before being recognized.

The fact that the disorder was associated with certain families, and that it could often be shown to affect succeeding generations, raised the interesting possibility that it might be inherited. One investigator felt that the scattered populations in which it had been discovered could have racial and genetic links. While these communities were now living in separate and distinct areas in three entirely different countries, all had a common heritage. They had all, in the past, belonged to a single great empire, the Ottoman Empire of Turkey.

A number of mass population migrations had certainly occurred within the Ottoman Empire. The Sopovi or Torlaci, for instance, had moved from their homelands in western Bulgaria and eastern Serbia, northwards along the valleys of the Morava and the Drina, leaving the districts where Balkan nephropathy was first discovered for the very regions where it was subsequently recognized. It was a curious accident of history that the Yugoslav village in which Balkan nephropathy was first discovered should have been called Sopici.

The most surprising part about it was that, while the Balkan nephropathy ignored modern political frontiers, the disorder was almost entirely confined within the boundaries of the old Ottoman Empire. Only at Slavonski Brod, where for centuries the River Sava defined the border between the Austrian and Turkish empires, did the disease cross the river to appear in a few isolated settlements on the northern bank. Yet even here place-names suggested a forced migration or flight from persecution. One settlement on the northern bank which harboured the disease was called Zbjeg, meaning 'refugee-shelter', and another was called Pricac, meaning 'crossing over the river'.

These historical speculations remained tenuous, however, as did the idea that intermarriage within secluded peasant communities might produce genetic predispositions to the disease. While cousin marriages were commonplace in Romania, in Bulgaria they had been forbidden on religious grounds even up to fourth-generation cousins. The difficulties with any genetic theory became apparent as soon as it was examined closely. For one thing, the disease was too successful. No inherited disorder has ever been seen to afflict such a large percentage of any population.

The best example of a proved 'epidemic' of a hereditary disease occurs among the Afrikaners in South Africa, where the porphyria gene, carried by one of the original Dutch settlers, still causes the disease in the descendants of old Dutch families. Among several million Afrikaners there are now several thousand cases of porphyria, but the incidence of porphyria in the Afrikaner population is still only approximately one in every thousand, or 0·1 per cent. By contrast, the incidence of Balkan nephropathy in some villages about Vratza ran as high as 12 per cent, and, if suspected cases were included, the figure rose to 40 per cent.

To add to the difficulties, many of the family trees which the investigators collected simply contained too many cases to be accounted for by a form of Mendelian inheritance. Furthermore, a long-term study made of identical twins, born in the endemic area but separated at an early age, showed that the ones who remained in the villages sometimes developed Balkan nephropathy while their twins who departed the region did not. Environment was evidently more important than inheritance.

The final blow to the genetic theory fell with the realization that the disease occasionally cropped up in individuals who, though they had lived in the district many years, had been born elsewhere: a woman who married into the farming community, for instance, or a labourer who moved into the district to take up permanent employment. A residence of at least fifteen years seemed necessary to qualify for catching the disease.

This fifteen-year residence before an outsider became liable was seized on, and two possible explanations were offered. The disease was either caused by some infection which had a very long incubation period or else by a very prolonged exposure to some poison or toxin present in the environment. Certain researchers even saw in the fifteen-year 'incubation' period an explanation for the rarity of the condition in childhood.

The Bulgarian authorities used a simple direct approach to take the matter further. In a determined, long-term experiment, all 113 inhabitants of the village of Karash in the Vratza region, where Balkan nephropathy was particularly severe, were persuaded to move to a new settlement outside the endemic area. The results were unequivocal. During the following ten years, forty-four of the uprooted villagers developed Balkan nephropathy in their new homes. Yet none of the children under fifteen at the time of the move developed the disease, nor did any children born subsequently. Five outsiders, who had been living in Karash for less than ten years at the time of the migration, also escaped unharmed.

By now various families had been traced who had migrated from the endemic regions of their own accord. Many of these had moved to such cities as Belgrade, Zagreb or Sarajevo, or even as far afield as Chicago or Stockholm. Some of them had then fallen sick with the Balkan nephropathy as long as ten or fifteen years after their move, but, as became increasingly clear, their children, who had spent all their lives in the towns, remained completely unaffected.

With the disease's tendency to produce several cases in a single household, it was natural to consider that it might be infectious. Yet there was no consistent evidence for bacterial infection to be found. Such micro-organisms as leptospira, brucella or streptococci, known to attack the kidney, were not found in these areas with any more frequency than they show in the rest of the world. They could not be isolated from patients, neither could the antibodies which an infection by them would have provoked be detected in patients' bloodstreams.

To counter these awkward aspects, it was suggested that the Balkan nephropathy might be the long-delayed end-result of a process initiated by a brief infection many years in the past. It would then be natural to expect that all traces of the original infection would have disappeared long before the patient came to be investigated. Against this ran the fact that no consistent histories of preceding illness could be obtained and that the pattern of kidney damage bore no marks of the inflammatory processes which would have inevitably been provoked by such a bacterial assault. The kidney changes indeed bore no resemblance to the end-results of any known bacterial infection.

One epidemiological curiosity lay in the fact that, although each country had a relatively large gypsy population – Bulgaria, for example, having at least 170,000 – these people seemed to enjoy an immunity even though they regularly visited the endemic regions and undertook casual work on the land. The investigators made the observation but, again, were utterly lost to explain it.

There were repeated attempts to incriminate a number of different viruses. Many villagers certainly lived in close proximity with pigs, and one research team favoured the pig coronavirus as their prime suspect. They formed the impression that, in the mixed populations which contained both Christians and Moslems, only Christians developed Balkan nephropathy. Moslems, they pointed out, did not eat pork or practice pig-husbandry. It was unfortunately not possible to confirm either the supposed immunity of Moslems or the presence of coronaviruses. Most attempts to implicate a virus were based on a hopeful identification of virus-like particles when kidneys from patients were examined under an electron microscope. No one was able to grow a viral type of culture from these particles, however, while it proved impossible to demonstrate viral antibodies in the patients.

Nevertheless the epidemiology of Balkan nephropathy was, with its greatly prolonged 'incubation' period, in many ways reminiscent of a characteristic slow-virus disease where the virus does not betray its presence in a victim for several years, revealing itself at last only through the development of a chronic progressive illness; and with a slow-virus infection, no viral antibody formation is provoked. Nevertheless all attempts to demonstrate a slow virus in Balkan nephropathy have so far failed.

With heredity and infection having to be dismissed as investigative dead-ends, the field was narrowed to the question of whether the disease was caused by a toxin or poison in the environment. All the endemic regions were, like Vratza, located on tributaries of the Danube and a consideration of the villagers' water supplies was therefore a natural line of inquiry. Almost all the villages in fact took their drinking-water from wells.

During its underground flow, water usually dissolves only minute quantities of the materials through which it passes. It is, however, possible that a dangerous concentration of some toxic substance could build up as a gradually accumulating hazard should the water be used regularly year after year. A bonus to this argument was that it seemed quite likely that water from the Danube flooded the ground-water and water-tables that supplied the wells in those villages which lay on the valley floors, while the wells in the unaffected villages at higher altitudes were fed directly by pure hill springs.

The theory was neat, but there were still snags. In Serbia, for instance, the town of Lazarevac, in which not a single case occurred, took its water from the same underground source as the village of Sopici, which was heavily affected. It was true that at Lazarevac the water was passed through only a simple treatment plant, but it seemed unlikely this would make much difference to the concentrations of substances carried. Analysis of the water in any case produced no results. No toxic substances could be found and the various trace elements were present only in concentrations that lay well within the limits set for drinking-water by the World Health Organization.

Investigations of diet proved to be just as indecisive. In the farming communities virtually all food was home produced. By Western standards, the staple diet was somewhat low in animal protein; many villagers ate meat only twice a week, and the researchers were amazed to find people who had not eaten animal protein for at least a month. Vegetables, fruit and grain were, however, plentiful. Mindful of catastrophes elsewhere, the investigators checked to see if seed grain treated with chemical pesticides was being consumed and what use was being made of artificial fertilizers and chemicals in growing crops. Yet it was already known that the disease must have existed long before the introduction of synthetic chemicals into agriculture.

When it came to traditional products, there were, curiously enough, no local cheeses, but most households distilled their own slivovitz, a brandy made from plums or other fruit. The drink contained a high concentration of copper since it was prepared and boiled in specially made copper vessels, but then this was a hazard borne equally by all slivovitz drinkers in the Balkan countries.

On the whole, diet seemed adequate, nutrition good, and it was impossible to detect any difference in the diets of those who had the disease and those who escaped, between affected and non-affected villages, or even between the endemic regions and the surrounding countryside. Plants were, however, not only used as vegetables, fruits or salads, but also as medicines. Most populations have their own folk-medicines and some herbal remedies have been shown to be dangerous. Could Balkan nephropathy therefore be caused by accidental vegetable poisoning?

The suggestion carried at least two favourable points. First, the recipes for such traditional remedies are often handed down within a family group, which would quite tidily explain the disease's tendency to occur within a household yet also appear in wives who married into it. Second, it could provide alternative but equally acceptable explanations for the greatly prolonged 'incubation' period. Under this hypothesis, Balkan nephropathy might arise either from a cumulative poisoning caused by years of ingesting repeated tiny doses of a toxic plant, or from a single dose of an extremely hazardous substance which took years to become apparent but eventually proved fatal; like certain alkaloids found in the 'diabetic cure' of a herbalist in Austria that had only needed one dose to inflict slow but inevitable and ultimately fatal damage. Moreover, it was vaguely suggested, perhaps the inhabitants of damp villages on valley floors had more need of household remedies for rheumaticky aches than those who lived higher up in the hills.

The initial problem with investigating the idea was that the local inhabitants tended to be guarded, protective and sometimes positively deceptive about their family remedies. The survey teams found themselves rebuffed, but it soon became apparent that a variety of so-called 'people's teas' was widely consumed. Infusions of herbs had for generations been used as medicines and abortifacients and even as virility aids. Such familiar local figures as village school teachers were enlisted to help compile collections of all the plants used as ingredients within each community. Discreet surveys then determined the remedies being used in each village or household. The study embraced both mountain-dwellers and plain-dwellers, both affected and unaffected households. Nevertheless the most determined efforts failed to detect any prevailing difference of disease between families who used 'people's teas' and families who did not.

Folk medicines were thus exonerated, but at least one dangerous plant was discovered growing in the area. This was Birthwort (*Aristolochia clematis*), which produces aristolochic acid, a substance capable of damaging the kidney in animals and man. It grows as a small weed in the cornfields of Eastern Europe and causes the passing of bloodstained urine in any animal unfortunate enough to eat it. Its recognition in the endemic areas led to the suspicion that bread made from grain contaminated by its seeds could be responsible. Mapping the distribution of birthwort in the fields of farmers whose families suffered from the disease produced no convincing links. More complex analytical studies were hampered by the acid and its metabolites being difficult to assay on any large scale, while the suggestions of critics simply pointed out that, in Yugoslavia at least, wheat grown in the endemic regions was distributed and used throughout the country.

Special studies of animal life brought to light several species of field and forest rodent previously unknown in the area, but it was impossible to identify any animal or insect which could act as a natural reservoir for some parasite capable of becoming a wholesale blight on the farming communities. There was also considerable curiosity about whether the disease could occur as well in domesticated animals. No evidence for it could be found in pigs, chickens, cows or ducks, but what looked like similar kidney damage was discovered in horses, dogs and cats, though it was very hard to state for certain that it was the same disease.

A human kidney is composed of about a million tiny filtering units called glomeruli, that filter water and such waste products as urea out of the bloodstream. From each tiny glomerulus the waste material is led down an elongated microscopic tubule which is looped into a shape faintly reminiscent of the convolutions of a trombone. Having traversed this minute tube, the waste material is drained into larger and larger collecting ducts which eventually empty it by way of the renal pelvis and ureter into the bladder. In many kidney diseases, the glomeruli bear the brunt of the damage. This is not so with the Balkan nephropathy. The disease is unusual in that it concentrates its attack on the renal tubules.

The renal tubule is more than a simple, if strangely shaped waste-pipe. It is an extremely efficient chemical inspection and adjustment department. Many of the substances which the glomeruli filter out are ones that the body can ill afford to lose in such quantities. These are therefore selectively reabsorbed by the tubule, while other products which have not been cleared sufficiently from the bloodstream are actively excreted into the flow of waste material. By a careful adjustment of the excretion and reabsorption of various ions and salts, the tubule in fact succeeds in balancing the chemical environment within the body. Since several substances are known to poison the renal tubule, it now made sense to check for them in Balkan nephropathy.

The most likely poison seemed to be one of the heavy metals. Cadmium, for instance, has caused a rather similar form of renal damage in Swedish workers exposed to it during an industrial process. Cadmium also occurs in certain soils and becomes deposited in plant tissues, and so can eventually find its way into food. Because it is excreted so very slowly (it has a biological 'half-life' of over thirty years), nearly all cadmium ingested is retained in the body. A North American on an average diet consumes about 80 micrograms of cadmium a day, and by the time the age of fifty is reached will have accumulated a concentration of between 10 and 40 micrograms of cadmium in every gram of kidney tissue. Only if this concentration should rise above 200 micrograms per gram will kidney damage set in.

The attractive hypothesis of cadmium poisoning faltered on the fact that the endemic regions of the Balkans offered no evidence for an excessive concentration of cadmium in either water or soil. It was found in Yugoslavia, on the other hand, that one of the most commonly used fertilizers contained ten to twenty times more cadmium than a similar phosphate fertilizer used in the United States. Plants grown under experimental conditions were found to contain at least ten times as much cadmium when nourished by the Yugoslav fertilizer, but the concentration was still far too low to produce significant disease even if eaten regularly over many years.

The arguments against cadmium seemed irrefutable. The Swedish victims of industrial exposure had suffered a similar kidney damage, but none of the victims had gone on to develop a chronic progressive renal failure. In Japan, where rice grown in water with a high cadmium content did cause widespread disease, this was characterized by a different clinical picture, one principally dominated by bone pains.

A different line of inquiry opened up in the Kolubara district of Serbia when research teams found approximately two and a half times the normal concentration of lead in flour being used by the farming communities. Their maize and wheat were, it emerged, being ground by a large water-mill that had eight grinding stones. The working surfaces of some of these mill wheels had grown worn and pitted, but, where these had been repaired, the indentations had been filled with a grey-brown mixture prepared by the miller himself. This home-made repair compound turned out to contain over 50 per cent of lead. As trials showed, the amount of lead in the grain was increased four-fold by the time it was ground into flour.

Unfortunately, several strong arguments existed against lead as the cause of Balkan nephropathy. To begin with, no evidence of excessive concentrations of lead could be discovered in any of the other endemic regions and the disease did not disappear from Serbia once the miller's unfortunate enterprise had been corrected. Secondly, the clinical picture of chronic lead poisoning, with blood pressure often being raised and urine heavily loaded with albumin, is well known and differs in certain important respects from that of Balkan nephropathy. Thirdly, apart from damaging the renal tubules, lead also attacks the glomeruli and renal blood vessels, changes not found in autopsies of patients with Balkan nephropathy. And finally, a standard treatment for removing lead from the body failed to produce any increased excretion of lead.

Yet another group of investigators sought to lay the blame on silicon, but silicon occurs widely throughout the world and, while it is known to damage the renal tubule, it has so far proved impossible to attribute to it any definite clinical symptoms. Furthermore, studies of water supplies in the endemic regions of Yugoslavia failed over ten years to reveal any abnormal concentrations of cadmium, lead or silicon, or, indeed, of any substance known to cause kidney damage. Attempts to incriminate radioactivity similarly showed that concentrations of radon, radium, thorium and uranium all fell within standard ranges.

Yet another important piece of the jigsaw was to emerge which was in many ways the most disconcerting piece of all. In only two of the three countries, Bulgaria and Yugoslavia, a second rare disease was discovered in exactly the same villages where Balkan nephropathy occurred. This second endemic was of a cancer, a malignant papilloma, a cauliflower-like tumour that grew from the linings of the passageways that led the urine from the kidney down to the bladder; in other words, from the walls of the renal pelvis and ureter. Technically, it was classified as a transitional-cell carcinoma. Like the nephropathy, it was rather more common in women than men and practically unknown in children; it hit almost exclusively at middle-aged members of the farming community.

Such tumours are known in practically every population in the world but remain rarities. In 1978, for instance, an observer commented that such a cancer had not been seen at the Cleveland County Metropolitan General Hospital during the previous decade. In Yugoslavia, the chances of a person living in Belgrade developing such a cancer were only about one in 20,000, while in Novi Sad the figure was as low as one in 45,000. Those who lived in the villages where Balkan nephropathy occurred, however, stood at least a one in 200 risk of developing this cancer.

In Bulgaria, a list of 104 women who had this form of cancer disclosed the startling fact that all but three of them lived in the endemic villages about Vratza. Just to rub the point in, it was then discovered that two of the remaining three had been born in villages in the endemic region and spent the first eighteen to twenty years of their lives there.

Nothing more was needed to emphasize the fact that the endemic regions featured an unusually high incidence of this malignant transitional-cell carcinoma, yet now it was found that many patients carried more than one such tumour. Whereas in Sweden only eighteen out of 10,682 patients with a cancer of the urinary tract were found to have multiple tumours, in the Vratza region, every third or fourth patient had at least two, three or even more of them.

Similar tumours were by now coming to light in the

endemic regions of the third country, Romania. It seemed an impossible coincidence that two rare diseases should occur in exactly the same scattered populations, attacking the same limited groups of people and displaying such comparable epidemiological features, unless they were in some way linked. The proof of a connection appeared to be shown by the fact that both diseases often occurred simultaneously in the same patient. A painstaking study in the Vratza region revealed that 35 per cent of patients with Balkan nephropathy featured one or more of these transitional-cell carcinomas. It was moreover found that 52 per cent of patients attending a surgical clinic in Belgrade with these tumours eventually died from uraemia, uraemia being a most unusual complication of tumours of the renal pelvis and ureter which would normally only be expected if tumour growth had obstructed the urine outflow from both kidneys or been accompanied by persistent disastrous kidney infections. Nearly all the tumour patients who died from uraemia were also suffering from Balkan nephropathy.

The recognition of these cancers in the endemic regions did, however, provide one much-needed clue. Several workers had suggested that mycotoxins, substances produced by fungi or moulds, should be investigated since mycotoxins already stood incriminated as the cause of various diseases in animals. It was now recognized that not only did some of them concentrate their attack on one specific organ of the body, but that one or two of them were also capable of stimulating the formation of unusual cancers. The fungus *Aspergillus flavus*, for example, which grows on ground-nuts, produces aflatoxin, a chemical which not only attacks the liver in animals but provokes the formation of rare liver tumours. No more than a single dose of aflatoxin is needed to set in train a steadily progressive liver disease.

Much research on mycotoxins had been carried out in Russia because of the damage which fungi infesting 'overwintered' grain had done to livestock. In Denmark, however, with its large pig industry, an interesting mycotic disease had been discovered in swine. Should pigs be allowed to feed upon rye or barley contaminated by the mould *Penicillium viridicatum*, they develop a kidney disease which bears some resemblance to Balkan nephropathy. As veterinary researchers discovered, the mould produced two substances called ochratoxin A and citrinin, which selectively attacked and destroyed a pig's renal tubules. Between 6 and 7 per cent of all Danish pigs' kidneys had to be condemned at slaughter.

It was an attractive hypothesis that a single mycotoxin could be responsible for both the Balkan nephropathy and the transitional-cell carcinomas. It was easy to see how the Balkans' hot Mediterranean summers and high humidity in the valley bottoms might combine to encourage the growth of moulds and fungi in crops. The Balkan villagers stored their grain in their *tavana* or house lofts, and a high moisture content in the grain would almost certainly lead to the development of moulds, especially of the *Penicillium* species; and it was strains of *Penicillium* which produced ochratoxin A and citrinin. The fungus might easily gain a permanent foothold in a loft, or even in a row of adjacent lofts, so explaining the tendency of the disease to occur over and over in one particular household.

If the theory continued to sound rather tentative, it had one remarkable observation to support it. The idea prompted a study of the weather, and almost at once a statistically significant correlation was discovered in the endemic regions between late summer and autumn rainfall and the numbers of local deaths from Balkan nephropathy in the succeeding two years. This has remained the only clear association discovered between any environmental factor and the incidence of the nephropathy.

The search was now on for ochratoxin A and citrinin in samples of 'over-wintered' grain, and research teams from Denmark helped not only to isolate ochratoxin A but to point out intriguingly that it was present in 12·8 per cent of grain samples from the endemic villages but only in 1·6 per cent of samples from outside the region. Furthermore, ochratoxin A was detected in pork from the area, and most significantly even in the blood of normal inhabitants from the endemic villages.

It was at this point that the chain of observations unfortunately broke apart. There were no indications of where the ochratoxin A came from; none of the various strains of *Penicillium* mould found in the area produced it. In an attempt to reforge the links, another team of researchers started at the opposite end of the puzzle by studying those mycotoxins produced by the fungi and moulds which could be identified in the endemic region. One mould in particular which caught their attention was *Penicillium verrucosum*. This, which usually grew on barley, was found in each of the different Balkan nephropathy areas. It was, in fact, the most commonly isolated species of fungi, being recovered from a wide variety of decaying vegetable matter, including mouldy garlic and maize, rotting quince, diseased paprika and fermenting plums. The mycotoxins produced by *Penicillium verrucosum* were not immediately identifiable, but they were shown to be capable of causing kidney damage to rats. Animals fed on mixtures containing the fungus developed an illness similar in many ways to Balkan nephropathy, the main injury being inflicted on the rats' renal tubules. Entirely lacking, however, was evidence to show that the fungus or its toxins was being consumed in any quantity by villagers as well as information about its effect on the human kidney.

Perhaps the most telling of numerous objections to the mycotoxin theory were based on simple epidemiology. *Penicillium verrucosum* was distributed widely throughout the world, yet Balkan nephropathy occurred only in highly restricted geographical areas. Although farmers in the endemic districts kept a high proportion of crops for their own use, surplus grain was sold week by week in the town markets and the town dwellers escaped unscathed.

The mycotoxin theory sought to explain the coexistence of Balkan nephropathy and transitional-cell tumours by supposing that the mycotoxin had a double action. The doctors themselves had been moving towards a neater explanation ever since it had been recognized quite early on that, unlike a vast majority of kidney disease sufferers, patients with Balkan nephropathy did not leak large quantities of albumin from the bloodstream into their urine. Their urine did contain a small quantity of protein, but this was of a much smaller molecule known as B-2-microglobulin; and B-2-microglobulin has been found in the urine of patients with other rare forms of kidney disease in which the renal tubule similarly bears the brunt of the attack. The presence of this protein in urine was, in fact, diagnostically regarded as a sensitive indication of damage to the renal tubules.

By devising methods of screening the urine of large numbers of people, it proved possible in the endemic villages to detect B-2-microglobulin in the urine of individuals who had as yet developed no clinical evidence of the disease. It was also present in young people, even in children as young as five years of age, though in these younger individuals B-2-microglobulin was found only intermittently. This suggested that the renal tubules were suffering minor but repeated episodes of damage. Presumably no full-blown clinical picture of Balkan nephropathy would emerge until a critical number of tubules were destroyed.

These discoveries were more or less predictable. The surprise came with the finding that patients with transitional-cell tumours also excreted B-2-microglobulin. It happened even in tumour patients where the most careful microscopic examination of kidney tissue failed to show the slightest trace of Balkan nephropathy. In other words, B-2-microglobulin was somehow as intimately connected with the presence of the endemic transitional-cell tumours as it was with the nephropathy itself. The expectation followed from this that both groups of patients would have B-2-microglobulin not only in the urine but also in raised levels in their blood-streams, and that the highest concentrations of all would be found in cells lining the renal tubules and in the substance of transitional-cell tumours.

This proved to be so, and the doctors intervened to offer their interpretation. In certain malignant diseases, such as acute leukaemia, there is just occasionally unmistakable evidence for a patient's renal tubules having been damaged, this seeming to be a chemical or toxic injury rather than a direct spread of a growth. The unusual explanation for this is that, in the malignant diseases where the complication occurs, the abnormal cancer cells produce large amounts of proteins of low molecular weight known as immunoglobulins. The kidney can then suffer damage when faced with having to clear low molecular weight proteins out of the bloodstream. While such a protein passes easily through the glomerulus or filter unit and is then reabsorbed in the first part of the renal tubule, the tubule can unfortunately only cope with small amounts. With higher concentrations, the cells lining the renal tubules become overloaded and damaged and unabsorbed protein precipitates into casts which block the tubule.

B-2-microglobulin was, it so happened, a protein of low molecular weight. From this there sprang the suggestion that the key to Balkan nephropathy lay not with renal tubules but with transitional-cell tumours. The hypothesis ran something as follows. The inhabitants of the endemic villages were exposed to some as yet unidentified toxin, possibly even a mycotoxin, which over the years provoked, first, a pre-cancerous and then a malignant change in the linings of the renal pelvis and ureter. As the cells lining these passageways became abnormal, they began to overproduce the low molecular weight protein B-2-microglobulin. This 'light chain' protein was then filtered from the bloodstream by the kidneys, in which process the renal tubules became overloaded and destroyed.

In contrast to such highly malignant diseases as acute leukaemia and multiple myeloma where the victim is swiftly overwhelmed, the transitional-cell carcinoma of the renal pelvis and ureter was a slow-growing tumour which almost never invaded other parts of the body. In the highly malignant, fast-moving conditions, a full clinical picture of kidney damage hardly had time to emerge. With a slow-growing transitional-cell tumour, however, the kidney disorder, which progressed quite rapidly, was often the first condition to declare itself and was thus likely to be seen as the dominant clinical illness, on many occasions totally eclipsing as yet undetected, microscopic cancerous changes in the walls of the urinary passages.

The hypothesis is neat and all-embracing. According to medical science, Balkan nephropathy is nothing more than a complication of transitional-cell tumours. But what has caused those tumours in the first place? The question of aetiology brings the inquiry back to square one and the pieces of the jigsaw lie on the table as unconnected as ever. More than thirty years of research, a series of symposia involving international experts and the publication of many learned articles have failed to produce an answer. Is it a mycotoxin? Is it an unrecognized contamination of water supplies? Is it, when all is said and done, a slow virus? Fresh minds, equipped by other philosophies, may be able to see what the medical scientists have missed. The facts are available; only the solution is lacking.

Selected Sources

CHAPTER 1: *The Stranded Eagle*

Andrée, S. A., Strindberg, Nils, and Fraenkel, Knut, *The Andrée Diaries: Being the Diaries and Records . . . Written during Their Balloon Expedition to the North Pole in 1897 and Discovered on White Island in 1930, together with a Complete Record of the Expedition and Discovery*, authorized translation from the official Swedish edition by Edward Adams-Ray, John Lane, The Bodley Head, London, 1931.

Kirwan, L. P., *A History of Polar Exploration*, Penguin Books, Harmondsworth, 1962. (Originally published as *The White Road*, Hollis and Carter, London, 1959.)

Rolt, L. T. C., *The Aeronauts: A History of Ballooning 1783–1903*, Longmans, London, 1966.

Roth, Hans, 'Nouvelles expériences sur la trichinose avec considérations spéciales sur son existence dans les régions arctiques', *Office international des épizooties: rapport à la XVIIIe session*, 1950, R: No. 174.

Roth, Hans, 'Trichinosis in Arctic Animals', *Nature*, 21 May 1949, pp. 805–6.

CHAPTER 2: *The Last Infirmity*

Bean, William E., *Walter Reed: A Biography*, University Press of Virginia, Charlottesville, 1982.

Kelly, H. A., *Walter Reed and Yellow Fever*, McClure Phillips, New York, 1906.

Woodward, Theodore E., 'Yellow Fever: From Colonial Philadelphia and Baltimore to the Mid-Twentieth Century', in Lilienfeld, Abraham M. (ed.), *Aspects of the History of Epidemiology*, Johns Hopkins University Press, Baltimore, 1980.

CHAPTER 3: *The Case of the Epping Jaundice*

Kopelman, H., Robertson, M. H., Sanders, P. G., and Ash, I., 'The Epping Jaundice', *British Medical Journal*, 26 February 1966, vol. I, pp. 514–16.
Kopelman, H., Scheuer, P. J., and Williams, R., 'The Liver Lesion of the Epping Jaundice', *Quarterly Journal of Medicine*, October 1966, vol. 35, pp. 553–64.

CHAPTER 4: *The Ghost Disease*

Farquhar, Judith, and Gajdusek, D. Carleton (eds.), *Kuru: Early Letters and Field-Notes from the Collection of D. Carleton Gajdusek*, Raven Press, New York, 1981.
Zigas, V., and Gajdusek, D. C., 'Kuru: Clinical Study of a New Syndrome Resembling Paralysis Agitans in Natives of the Eastern Highlands of Australian New Guinea', *Medical Journal of Australia*, 23 November 1957, pp. 745–54.

CHAPTER 5: *Death in the Parish*

Chave, S. P. W., 'Henry Whitehead and Cholera in Broad Street', *Medical History*, vol. II, no. 2, 1958, pp. 92–108.
Longmate, Norman, *King Cholera: The Biography of a Disease*, Hamish Hamilton, London, 1966.
Minutes of the Vestry of St James, Westminster, MS in the Westminster City Archives.
Report on the Cholera Outbreak in the Parish of St James, during the Autumn of 1854, Presented to the Vestry by the Cholera Inquiry Committee, July 1855, Churchill, London, 1855.
Snow, John, *On the Mode of Communication of Cholera*, second edition, Churchill, London, 1855.
Whitehead, Rev. H., 'The Broad Street Pump: An Episode in the

Cholera Epidemic of 1854', *Macmillan's Magazine*, December 1865, pp. 113–22.

CHAPTER 6: *A Fallen Splendour*

'Arsenic in the House', annotation, *Lancet*, 28 July 1956, pp. 182–3.
'Arsenical Poisoning, The Work of the Swedish Committee', *Lancet*, 5 September 1923, pp. 531–2.
Shadegg, Stephen, *Clare Boothe Luce*, Leslie Frewin, London, 1973.
Sheed, Wilfred, *Clare Boothe Luce*, Weidenfeld and Nicolson, London, 1982.
The Times, 18, 19, 20 and 23 July 1956.
Time Magazine, 23 July 1956, p. 11.

CHAPTER 7: *The Visitor from a Far Country*

Brown, Herbert H., 'The Recent Plague Cases in Suffolk', *British Medical Journal*, 12 November 1910, p. 1490.
Gregg, Charles T., *Plague! The Shocking Story of a Dread Disease in America Today*, Charles Scribner's Sons, New York, 1978.
Sleigh, H. P., 'Four Cases of Pneumonic Plague', *British Medical Journal*, 12 November 1910, pp. 1489–90.
Zwanenberg, David Van, 'The Last Epidemic of Plague in England? Suffolk 1906–1918', *Medical History*, vol. XIV, no. 1, January 1970, pp. 62–74.

CHAPTER 8: *The Paradoxes of a Small American Disaster*

Silverman, William A., *Retrolental Fibroplasia: A Modern Parable*, Grune and Stratton, New York, 1980.
Stark, D. J., Manning, L. M., and Lenton, L., 'Retrolental Fibroplasia Today', *Medical Journal of Australia*, 21 March 1981, pp. 275–80.

CHAPTER 9: *The Beetle of Aphrodite*

'Cantharidin Poisoning', editorial, *British Medical Journal*, 11 December 1954, pp. 1405–6.

Craven, J. D., and Polak, A., 'Cantharidin Poisoning', *British Medical Journal*, 11 December 1954, pp. 1386–8.
Gorer, Geoffrey, *The Life and Ideas of the Marquis de Sade*, revised edition, Panther, London, 1964.
Heine, M., 'L'affaire des bonbons cantharidés du Marquis de Sade', *Hippocrate*, vol. I, 1933, pp. 95–133.
Nickolls, L. C., and Teare, D., 'Poisoning by Cantharidin', *British Medical Journal*, 11 December 1954, pp. 1384–6.'
Oaks, W. W., et al., 'Cantharidin Poisoning', *American Medical Association Archives of Internal Medicine*, vol. 105, 1960, pp. 575–82.

CHAPTER 10: *The Contagion and the Rose*

Fitzgerald, James A., 'Rosebush Scratch', *New York State Journal of Medicine*, 1 May 1972, pp. 1077–80.
Graham, Harvey, *Eternal Eve*, William Heinemann Medical Books, London, 1950.
Holmes, Oliver Wendell, 'The Contagiousness of Puerperal Fever', originally published in the *New England Quarterly Journal of Medicine and Surgery*, vol. 1, 1843, and 'Puerperal Fever as a Private Pestilence', originally published as a pamphlet by Ticknor and Fields, Boston, Mass., 1855; both reprinted in *Medical Classics*, vol. I, no. 3, November 1936.
Jewett, John Figgis, Reid, Duncan E., Safon, Leonard E., and Easterday, Charles L., with a comment by Watson, Benjamin, 'Childbed Fever – A Continuing Entity', *Journal of the American Medical Association*, vol. 206, no. 2, 7 October 1968, pp. 344–50.

CHAPTER 11: *The Head that Wore a Crown*

Chalmers, Rev. Peter, *A Historical and Statistical Account of Dunfermline*, 2 vols., William Blackwood and Sons, Edinburgh and London, 1844.
Møller-Christensen, Vilhelm, 'Cases of Leprosy and Syphilis in the Osteological Collection of the Department of Anatomy, University of Edinburgh', *Danish Medical Bulletin*, 1963, pp. 175–83.
Møller-Christensen, Vilhelm, *Leprosy Changes of the Skull*, Odense University Press, 1978.

'The Skull of Robert the Bruce', *Medical Journal and Record*, vol. 121, 1925, pp. 643–4.

CHAPTER 12: *The Walk to Eternity*

Cleland, Sir John, and Southcott, R. V., 'Hypervitaminosis A in the Antarctic in the Australasian Antarctic Expedition of 1911–1914: A Possible Explanation of the Illnesses of Mertz and Mawson', *Medical Journal of Australia*, 28 June 1969, pp. 1337–42.

Kirwan, L. P., *A History of Polar Exploration*, Penguin, Harmondsworth, 1962. (Originally published as *The White Road*, Hollis and Carter, London, 1959.)

Mawson, Sir Douglas, MS Diaries in the Mawson Institute of Antarctic Research, University of Adelaide, Australia.

Mawson, Sir Douglas, *The Home of the Blizzard; Being the Story of the Australasian Antarctic Expedition, 1911–1914*, vol. I, Heinemann, London, 1915.

Rodahl, K., and Moore, T., 'The Vitamin A Content and Toxicity of Bear and Seal Liver', *Biochemical Journal*, vol. 37, 1943, p. 166.

Southcott, R. V., Chesterfield, N. J., and Lugg, D. J., 'Vitamin A Content of the Livers of Huskies and Some Seals from Antarctic and Sub-Antarctic Regions', *Medical Journal of Australia*, 6 February 1971, pp. 311–13.

CHAPTER 13: *The Balkan Enigma*

Austwick, Peter K. C., in the *Practitioner*, vol. 225, July 1981, pp. 1031–8.

Hall, Philip W., III, and Damin, G. J., 'Balkan Nephropathy', *Nephron*, vol. 22, 1978, pp. 281–300.

Wolstenholme, G. E. W., and Knight, J. (eds.), *The Balkan Nephropathy*, Ciba Foundation Study Group, No. 30, 1967.

Index